MW00860758

PATANJALI YOGA SUTRAS
पतांजली योग सुत्र

A Commentary by
H. H. Sri Sri Ravi Shankar

Volume 1

ARKTOS
LONDON 2014

Patanjali Yoga Sutras - Volume 1
A Commentary by H. H. Sri Sri Ravi Shankar

1st Edition, September 2010, Sri Sri Publications Trust, Bangalore
2nd Edition, January 2014, Arktos Media Ltd., London

Printed in the United Kingdom.

ISBN **978-1-907166-35-8**

BIC classification:
Mind, Body, Spirit: thought and practice (VXA)
Mind, body, spirit: meditation and visualisation (VXM)
Hinduism (HRG)

ARKTOS MEDIA LTD
www.arktos.com

Contents

Chapter 1

DISCIPLINE OF YOGA

अथ योगानुशासनम्

Atha yogaanushaasanam.

Shaasana are the rules that society or somebody else imposes on you. *Anushaasana* are the rules that you impose on yourself.

Now, why is Yoga called a discipline?

Where is the need for a discipline?

When does the need for a discipline arise?

When you are thirsty, you want to drink water. You do not feel that it is a rule to drink water when you are thirsty. And when you are hungry you eat. You do feel that you have the discipline of eating when you are hungry; that you have a discipline of enjoying the nature. No discipline is necessary for enjoyment. When is discipline relevant? Not when something is enjoyable at the very first step. A child never says that it has the discipline of running to his mother when he sees her.

Discipline arises where something is not very charming to begin with; when you know that it would ultimately give a fruit that is very good and enjoyable but that, in the beginning, it is not enjoyable. When you are abiding in yourself, when you are in joy, and when you are in peace or happiness, true happiness, then you are already in your Self. There is no discipline there. But when that is not so, the mind will wag its tail all the time. Then, discipline is essential to calm it down so that it can come back to it Self. The fruit of this is eventually blissful and joyful. A diabetic patient has a discipline not to eat sugar. Someone with cholesterol has to be disciplined and not take too much fat. This is because, though fats are tasty, they will raise unpleasant complications later.

There are three types of happiness – *sattvic, tamasic and rajasic.*

Sattvic, to begin with, is not so enjoyable but it always leads to joy. The happiness which is felt after a certain discipline is really *sattvic* happiness – a long lasting happiness. A happiness which is enjoyable to begin with, but ends in misery is no happiness at all. So, a discipline is necessary to have this authentic *sattvic* happiness. Discipline is not torturing oneself unnecessarily. The purpose of discipline is to attain joy.

Sometimes people impose disciplines on themselves which does not give any joy to them or to anybody else at any time.

This is *tamasic* happiness. *Tamasic* happiness just appears to be so but it is misery from the beginning to the end. No discipline is necessary for *tamasic* happiness. Lack of discipline is *tamasic* happiness.

Rajasic happiness appears very enjoyable in the beginning but ends up in misery and suffering. It is caused by following the wrong discipline. It may also arise from a lack of discipline.

Discipline is essential for *sattvic* happiness. To bear what is uncomfortable is discipline. It need not be uncomfortable all the time. But if it is uncomfortable, you need discipline to be able to bear it and move through it.

That is why Patanjali began with "Now" –when things are not clear and when your heart is not in the right place.

Yogaanushaasanam - Nobody has imposed the discipline of Yoga on you. They are self-imposed. What are the rules that you have imposed on yourself? When you wake up in the morning, you brush your teeth. You do it before going to bed, too. This is your discipline. But this has been imposed on you from childhood. When you were a kid, your mother had imposed it on you. Once it became a habit and when you understood that it was good for you, it was no more you mother's rule. It became your rule. Keeping yourself clean and observing hygiene, exercising, meditating, being kind, considerate, and not being rude - you have imposed these rules on yourself to help maintain your discipline.

Now, what does discipline do?

Discipline unites your Self and unites all the loose ends of your existence.

तदा द्रष्टुः स्वरूपेऽवस्थानम्

Tadaa drashtuh swaroopae avasthaanam.

It puts you on to your Self. *Tadaa drishta swaroopae avasthaanam.*

Otherwise, what has been happening?

वृत्ति सारूप्य मितरत्र

Vritti swaroopaya mitaratra.

Your mind has been engaged and caught up in the outside world all the time. Your eyes have been open and you have been caught up in all that you have been seeing. Similarly, you have been caught up in all that you smell, hear, touch, taste, etc. And when you are awake, you are constantly engaged in the activities of the senses. Otherwise, you go back to sleep and dream. Then, you are completely shut off.

During sleep and dream, the same memories come but you are never calm and quiet. When you unite all the loose ends of your existence, you become the object of your perception. When simple people or children watch a movie, they become totally involved in it. At that time, nothing else exists - just the movie. If you have a backache or a pain in your legs or back, it will seem more intense if you are idle. But when you are engaged in watching a movie then you do not feel the pain or anything else. You do not feel your body at all. You are not even aware that you are sitting. That is the deep interest the movie has aroused in you. Your consciousness has assumed the form of that movie, of that *vritti*.

Once, the people were watching a movie in a village. They saw that the hero was being tortured by the villain. The audience actually rushed towards the screen with sticks and stones, saying that they would hit the villain.

A great reformist of India was watching a drama, and the villain acted very well. This gentleman actually threw his shoe at him because he was so mad at him. He asked the villain how he could be so bad. The actor took it all as a compliment. He said that his acting was so good and he could captivate him so much with it that he actually threw his shoe at him.

Our consciousness assumes the form.

The whole purpose of Yoga is to be unto one Self - to bring integrity in you and to make you whole. You may be looking at me. Then, become aware of your eyes which are looking at me. And become aware of the mind that is looking at me through those eyes. Now for a moment close your eyes. Just squeeze them. Feel your eyes and take your attention from the eyes to the mind that is all over your head. Now, become aware of your whole body, your heart and the very core of your existence – the "I" that is you. Rest and relax there, right there. Then, you are not interested in seeing anything, smelling anything, hearing anything, or tasting anything, or feeling, or touching anything. Retrieve your mind from all the five senses, to the core of your heart or your existence. This is *drishtuhu swaroopae avasthaa.* Abiding there in the form of the seer is Yoga. Abiding in that form in the nature of the seer is Yoga. You are abiding in the form and the nature of the seer, knowingly or unknowingly, whenever you experience joy, ecstasy, bliss, or happiness in life. Otherwise, at other times, you are involved in and attached to the different activities of your mind.

Vritti swaroopae mitaratra. You assume the form in the mind. What are the activities in the mind?

Vrittayah panchatayyaha.

The modulations of the mind are of five forms – *klishta* and *aklishta.*

Some are problematic, and some are non-problematic. There are certain *vrittis* of the mind which are problematic and which cause troubles and difficulties, and certain others which are not problematic - unpleasant and pleasant *vrittis.*

Pramaana, viparyaya, vikalpa, nidraa and smritayaha.

Five modes of consciousness arise in you - five modes in the mind. Mind, consciousness or *chitta* are the same.

Pramaana, the mind is engaged in wanting proof for everything. There are three types of *pramana* – *pratyaksha, anumaana, aagamana.*

Pratyaksha means that which is obvious or can be experienced. You may be in Switzerland. You have a proof of this in your mind. The proof is that you can see the Swiss Alps. Whatever you see is a proof. You know that you are feeling cold. Nobody needs to tell you that. This is *pratyaksha*. Our mind constantly wants to have some obvious, solid or experiential proof. This is one mode of activity of the mind.

Another is *anumaana*. It means something which is not so obvious, but which can be guessed. You will believe in whatever you guess. The guessing of the mind is called *anumaana*.

Then there is *aagamana*, the scriptures. They are believed because they are written. These are the three types of proof you look for. Even today in certain remote villages, in the third world countries, anything that is printed is the gospel truth. People feel that, since many follow it, it must be the truth. A few people can be fooled in this way but not many. The mind feels that thousands are not fools. And if they are, then the mind feels that it can also be a fool. The mind works this way. It takes proof from scriptures or from the belief of many. *Aagamana pramaana.* You are constantly looking for proof of something or anything. This is one mode of activity.

Yoga is when you drop this. Then alone can you abide in the Self. Retreating from this activity of the mind of wanting proof is being released from that *vritti,* or activity of the mind, and going back to the Self. You may need proof of whether you are in Switzerland and your senses will tell you that. But you do not need proof, through your senses, whether you are where you are currently. You could be taken to Austria or to Canada. You will see similar snowy mountains and lakes there. You may think that you are in Switzerland but you are not. Your senses may fool you. But the feeling of "I am and I exist" is beyond proof.

Abiding in the Self does not need proof. Truth cannot be understood through proof. Anything that can be proved can also be disproved. Truth is beyond proof or disproof. God is beyond proof. You can neither prove God, nor can you disprove Him. Proof is connected with logic, and logic is very limited in its purview. It is the same with enlightenment and with love. Love cannot be proved or disproved. Someone's actions and behaviour is not a proof of love. Many movie actors and actresses exhibit a lot of love and romance in the movie but they need not experience real love or romance. They can just display it. One can act the emotion of love very well without feeling it or living it. Self is beyond all this proof. Proof is one of the main activities of the mind.

Proof is one of the main things that you are stuck with in this world. You want proof for everything. This is not in the realm of the seer. A seer is beyond proof. *Pramaana* is the first modulation or activity of the mind.

Then comes *viparyaya*.

Patanjali describes this very beautifully in each of these modulations.

विपर्ययो मिथ्याज्ञानमतद्रूपप्रतिष्ठम्

Viparyayo mithyaa gyanam atad roopa pratishtham.

Pramaana is the knowledge that the mind is constantly engaged in arguments, in proofs, in knowledge, in analysing, or in wrong knowledge, wrong understanding, etc. You could be arguing and being logical. You could be looking for proof, or you will have wrong understanding. You will think things are the way that they are not. Most of the time you impose your own views, ideas, and feelings on others. You think that this is how the things are. This activity of mind is called *viparyaya*. You may have an inferiority complex and, thereby, consider someone's behaviour very arrogant. Actually, they are not arrogant, and you are not being ill-treated by them. But, you feel that you are being ill-treated. You feel that you have not been respected. It is because you do not respect yourself enough that you think that the others do not respect you. This tendency of your mind is *viparyaya*.

Others will be shocked by the change in your behaviour. They will wonder what has happened to you.

A very good friend of yours suddenly starts being very rude to you and you wonder what has happened to him. You wonder what it is that you have done to cause this. You do not understand that they are imagining things about you in their minds. It is not because they are bad or anything. It is this activity of the *chitta*, of the mind becoming predominant.

Suddenly, people may feel that they are not being loved. Many parents have this problem with their children. They get so perplexed. They do not know what to do and how to prove their love to their children. Proof is of no importance once *viparyaya* dominates. The *pramaana* does not survive, and logic fails because the mind is now more active on the second modulation, the second *vritti*, that is *viparyaya*. Only incorrect information sticks on. The correct knowledge appears briefly somewhere in their minds but returns to the background again, and the wrong information sticks on.

Mithyaa jnanam atad roopa pratishtam. This is *viparyaya*.

The third *vritti* is *vikalpa*.

Vikalpa is a sort of hallucination. There may be some thought. But, it is not true. However, something hovers in the mind. This is called *vikalpa*. People become paranoid. All such unfounded and baseless fears do not mean anything. Such thoughts and ideas are called *vikalpas* - fantasies. The mind either get stuck in proof or in wrong knowledge, misconceptions or fantasies. Fantasies are *vikalpa*. You may be already forty, fifty or sixty years old, and you fantasize what it would be like if you were sixteen again. Then, you go on and think that you would go somewhere and get a big haul of gold and that, then, you would become rich. Then, you would have your own helicopter to fly in. It is not just the children who fantasize. Adults also get into their own fantasies. This fantasy is called *vikalpa*, the third modulation of *chitta*.

Vikalpa could be of two types. One could be of just a joyful and pleasurable fantasy, and the other could be baseless fears. Even fear is a *vikalpa*. You may be apprehensive about what will happen if you die the next day. You may meet with an accident. You may become disabled. These are all just sounds that have no value. Baseless fears in the mind or fantasies are called *vikalpa*.

The fourth one is *nidra* or sleep. If the mind is not in any one of the three *vikalpas*, then it is asleep.

The fifth activity of the mind is *smriti* - remembering the experiences it has had. When you are awake, are you in any of these four states of modulations? Then, that is not meditation. That is not Yoga.

Are you looking for some proof? Are you debating with yourself? Are you hanging on to the wrong knowledge or concepts about how things are? You do not know how things are because the whole world is fluid. There is nothing solid here. Nobody is solid. Nobody's mind is solid. No thoughts are solid. The whole world is fluid or even airy. Go one step further, and you can say it is all airy-fairy! Anything can change at anytime and in any manner. The whole world is full of probabilities and possibilities. But your mind gets fixed on things, people, ideas, places, etc. It categorizes them into definite items, quantities, etc. This is how it is - set ideas, using the proof of the wrong information or the *vikalpa*, fantasizing and dwelling in the past experiences. The four modulations of mind plus the sleep, the fifth modulation, are the five different *vrittis* of the mind.

अभ्यासवैराग्याभ्यां तन्निरोधः

Abhyaasa vairagyaabhyaam tan nirodhah.

How will you get over the overpowering nature of these *vrittis*?

It is through *abhyasa* and *vairagya* – practice and detachment.

तत्र स्थितौ यत्नोऽभ्यासः

Tatra sthithau yatno abhyaasaha.

That which you do to 'be' is called *abhyasa* or practice. Abiding in the seer is *abhyasa*. That which you do to be there, now, here or in this moment is *abhyasa*. An effort is needed for you to relieve yourself from the five modulations and just be here – now, now, now; to bring the mind to the present and not dwell on past memories. This effort is called *abhyasa*.

You can start by being determined that you are not going to dwell on any logic. You are free from *pramaana*. You are not going to be interested in any proof. If the mind is asking for proof, just know it. Know it, observe it and relax. You are not interested in any wrong knowledge or right knowledge. Often when the mind is on wrong knowledge, it thinks it is on the right one. So, it is not even interested in knowing anything. Retrieve the mind from knowing, and from knowledge. There is no anxiety to see, smell, touch, feel or understand anything. Let things be the way they are. Do not care. Do not pass judgements of right or wrong. Free yourself from *viparyaya*, v*ikalpa*. Check if the mind is on some imagination or some fantasy. By just knowing that it is imagining or fantasizing, it drops off. It is just like the time when you know that you are dreaming - the dream vanishes. Knowing you are on a *vikalpa*, or a fantasy, it just drops off, thereby freeing you. This moment is so new, so fresh and so total. A*bhyasa* is just recognizing the moment when you are free, fresh, full and totally in the present moment. Here your mind might try to go into the past. You know that the mind is getting into the five *vrittis* without any aversion or craving. This is coming back to the centre; to the seer.

This moment, again and again and again, is *abhyasa*.

Chapter 2

HONOURING THE PRACTICE

Never mind. The mind can never go where you are. A wave can never go to the depth of the ocean. By the time the wave goes to the depth, it ceases to be a wave. So the mind can never come to you. The mind can never be you. That is why never mind! You are never the mind. It is superficial. The moment that mind starts coming towards you, it is not a mind. That is why it is said, "Never mind." You are accepted there; never the mind. Your mind can never go there.

You know you have had this experience often. The mind keeps on asking questions, "Why, why, why, why?" You feel that something that is bothering you is your mind's stuff! At that moment there is alertness, and an awareness dawns. And then there is a relief in the mind. And the more you feel that your questions are just "mind's stuff!", more and more you are aware. And then, the questions just vanish. This is *abhyaasa*, this is practice.

In the next sutra, Patanjali says,

स तु दीर्घकालनैरन्तर्यसत्कारासेवितो दृढभूमिः

Sa tu dheerghakaala nairantharya sathkaara sevito dridha bhoomih.

The effort to be still and steady comes with practice. At some time you may realize that it is the moment. And then it vanishes. You feel that the moment had come and you lost it. You say, "Now," and then the "Now" is lost. It may not be right to say you have lost it but, in some sense, you feel you are not in the "Now." But, this effort is not just linear –this effort to be steadily established in the "Now" because of it. The "Now" is not linear. The "Now" is very deep and vast. The "Now", the present moment, is not just a point; not just a dot. It is infinity. It is "Now" in all dimensions and from all sides. Practice gives stability in that moment – that is the purpose of practice. And how can that be arranged? How can that be achieved?

Sa tu dheergakaala – it takes a long time. *Nairantharya* means without a gap. *Sathkaara sevita* means with honour and respect - receiving it and practicing it with honour and respect. *Dhrida bhoomi* – then it becomes firmly established. Anything of value in life takes some time to culture. To master an art - cooking, playing a guitar, sitar, or a flute - takes some time. You cannot learn to play the flute in a day. It is not possible. To learn to play an instrument takes quite a while, and to master it even more. A coach is needed to teach how to play football. If you want to be a sportsman, you need a coach and you need practice. You need a coach in a gymnasium. You cannot make your body muscular overnight. It takes quite a long time. The body has its own requirement of time for its growth. Similarly, the mind takes even longer for its growth. It takes some time to memorize something. In the same way, any practice takes some time. It need not be too long but sufficiently long and without interruption. We usually learn something for a time and then stop. We will start again after some time. If we feel like doing it, we do, and don't do it if we do not want to; when we feel a little lazy. Then, the connection is broken, and what we want does not happen. Constant practice without a gap is essential. If you go to the gymnasium for a couple of days and stop and then go again after some time, you will not achieve anything. You may practice on the piano for two days and lay off for two months. Then, you start playing again. There is no consistency and nothing is gained. Lack of consistency prevents you from learning any art.

Therefore, *sa tu dheergakaala* – a long time without a gap. *Sathakara sevita.* - This is another important point – with honour and respect. Sometimes, we grumble when we do something. It is of no use doing something unenthusiastically. That is not *abhyasa. Abhyasa* is something done with gratitude, gratefulness, honour and with respect. This is something we lack in our life. We should do everything in life with honour and respect. Even if you do something with honour and respect, it lasts a very short period. And, if you have to do something over a period of time, you tend to lose that honour and respect. If you have to arrange a stage and, if you are doing it for the first time, you will do it with all honour and respect. You will put in so much attention, so much love, so much heart and awareness. But if you have to do it everyday for the next five to six months, you will just do it without the spirit with which you did on the first day. As time goes on, you seem to lose that alertness, attention, attentiveness, and honour. You feel wonderful the first day when you sit for meditation because you are doing it with all honour. But after some sessions you will feel bored by it. You will just sit and close your eyes. It does not have the same effect.

If any day, your meditation or *Kriya* is a little low, it is because you have lost respect for it; not that you disrespect it, but the attentiveness and alertness towards it is reduced. When you come together in a course, periodically, your meditation is deeper because you are receiving it with honour. You are honouring that knowledge. You are honouring yourself.

What is honour and honouring? Have you ever thought about it? Honour is total attentiveness to the present moment, with a tinge of gratefulness. If you honour a mountain, it means that you are seeing the mountain with all your heart and mind - without questioning or without debating within yourself. You are just honouring, being happy and grateful for what the mountain is. You honour some Nobel scientist. What does this mean? When the Nobel scientist is there, you are completely in the moment, being with that moment with all your heart – respecting and honouring.

Respect and honour every moment of your life. Then that becomes a practice. You respect your own body. That is practice; the *asanas*. What are *Asanas*? *Asanas* are respecting your own body consciously every moment. Respecting and honouring your breath and keeping it up over a period of time is *pranayam*. This is just like *Kriya* and the dimensions in *Kriya*. What is needed here is that you have to do the *Kriya* with the rhythm. Any practice is a practice only if it is done over a period of time – respectfully and without a gap. It is a practice only if you honour it every day and every moment. Then it becomes firmly established. This is very vital!

Any day when you feel that your meditation has become dull, check if you have kept up the continuity of the practice. If you feel that you have, then check if you have been honouring the mantra and the chanting time; if you have been honouring the life in you. If any one of these is not being followed, then your meditation will go haywire. So, determine to honour. Consider all the other events to be trivial. Just honour the moment. It is very precious. However the moment may be, it is very precious.

Honour the word. A Master has given you the word. It is so precious. Honouring the Master is honouring the Master's word. If you do not have honour or respect for the Master, your meditation will not work. This is because that honour and the respect awakens the consciousness and raises awareness in you. It helps you to focus on the moment totally. If you do not honour the Master, the Master will not lose anything. Your own mind will lose because it will be unable to be in the moment totally and to dive deep into the Source.

Sathkara sevita - honouring; honouring the source of knowledge, honouring the Master, honouring the knowledge, honouring the receiver.

A good musician will honour the music, and the one who has taught him and the one who composed it. His full attention is there. It is the same with a good sportsman. He will honour his coach. If he does not honour his coach, he will not progress. Due to his attentiveness and the honour that he has for the coach, he is able to move ahead in his sports. Otherwise, if he keeps judging his coach and does what he wants to, then what is the need for a coach? This is *abhyasa*, the practice.

Is this enough? Is just the *abhyasa*, the practice enough? No, it is not. There are two oxen that are needed to pull this cart. One is *abhyasa* and the other is *vairagya*.

What is *vairagya*?

दृष्टानुश्रविकविषयवितृष्णस्य वशीकारसंज्ञा वैराग्यम्

Drishta anushravika vishaya vitrishnasya vashikaara sangya vairagyam.

Drishta anushravika vishaya – The mind gallops towards the world of five senses. If you just be quiet, close your eyes, or open your eyes, or do anything, where does your mind go? It goes towards the sense of sight. It is the same for the sense of smell, taste, sound, touch. And this craving for any of these experiences in the mind can prevent you from being in the present moment.

Vairagya is retrieving your senses from the craving or from the thirst for something back to its source for a few moments. Then, you will feel that however beautiful a scene is, you are not interested in looking at it. However great the food, you feel that it is not the time for it; that you are not interested in tasting it then. However melodious the music maybe, you do not want to listen to it at that time. It may be wonderful to touch something but then you are not interested in touching it or feeling it at that time. *Vairagya* may be present for even a few moments. This is another basic requirement for meditation. This dispassion has to arise in your mind whenever you want to do meditation - a deep meditation. Without dispassion, your meditation is no good. It is of no use. It cannot provide you the rest that you are longing for.

Your mind is tired and burnt out because of its galloping on towards desires after desires. Just look back and check all the desires that you have achieved. Have they given you rest? They have not. They have just created a few more desires in you. Have they given you any fulfilment? They have not. They have just given you a greater hope that you can achieve more; that you can have more. And that has sent you on another pointless trip. You are on a merry-go-round. It is not even a merry-go-round. It just goes round and round. A merry-go-round has dummy horses which you sit on. The horses do not go anywhere. They just go round and round in the same place, but give you an illusion that you have travelled miles and miles – an illusion because you have reached nowhere. Life has been such a journey where you are galloping, galloping and galloping and reaching nowhere. This is what desires do for you. The mind which is obsessed with desires cannot meditate.

There are two types of attitudes. Some people feel that the mind should not have any desires and this becomes another desire. Destroy the desires. Some people are on this trip to destroy their desires. They are beating around the bush. Nothing happens to them. This principle should be very well understood.

Vitrushnasya vashikaara. The craving for any of the sense objects or celestial or heavenly places that the mind gallops towards is an obstruction. Any expectation in meditation is an obstruction. You may have heard that someone had seen a light or somebody coming from heaven and taking them by hand. So, you sit with your eyes closed and wait for an angel to come or to have a light shine on you and then to burst into a million stars. All these ideas and thoughts become an obstruction.

If you have dispassion, you will feel that you are not giving up anything for any of these pleasures. Your desire for pleasure or happiness will make you unhappy. If you examine yourself whenever you are miserable or unhappy, you will find that the misery is due to your desire to be happy. Craving for happiness brings misery. If you do not even crave for happiness, you are happy. You crave for happiness and you invite misery. When you do not care for happiness, you are liberated and when you do not even care for liberation, you attain love. This is *param vairagya*. But that is the second step. The first step is when you do not care for happiness. Then you are free. You are liberated.

Happiness is a mere idea in your mind. You think if you have something, you will be happy. If you have whatever you want, are you happy? Then, you will think it was not the way that you had thought it would be.

Vairagya is putting a stop to the craving for happiness.

This does not mean you have to be miserable. It does not say you should not enjoy. But if you can retrieve your mind from the craving for joy, you can meditate. Then, you can still all the five modulations, and Yoga happens.

You need to shatter all your dreams and fantasies. Offer them to the fire. Burn them down. What great happiness do you want? How long can you have it? You are going to leave this life at some time or the other. This is certain. It is all going to end. Before this earth eats you up, become free. Free yourself from the feverishness that is gripping your mind. Free yourself from the craving for happiness. What great happiness are you having? Every object of pleasure that you have experienced will become like Styrofoam, the packing material – absolutely tasteless!

You should study every craving that you have and remember that you are going to die. You may have a craving for sweets, sugar, food, etc. Have the craving and check consciously what is in it. You will find that there is nothing. You may crave for beautiful scenes. Keep looking at them. How long can you look? Your eyes will get tired of even the most beautiful place. Then, you will close them. You will forget the scenes. What other craving can come up in you – sex? How much sex can you have? Have it and finish it. You will see there is nothing in it. A few moments of it and that body, which was so attractive, looks like Styrofoam.

All these objects that titillate the senses have their limitations. But your mind is not ready to accept these limitations. It wants unlimited joy and pleasure which the five senses cannot give you. You simply get burnt down going over and over the same thing.

Vairagya is skillfully coming on to the Self by honouring all the objects of senses and not blaming them. This is dispassion - *vairagya*. Often, people who think they have dispassion keep blaming the world and the objects of senses. They are afraid of objects of senses and try to run away from them. They think that they are big temptations. The fear of temptations is worse. How can something tempt you?

This is the second sutra-

तत्परं पुरुषख्यातेर्गुणवैतृष्ण्यम्

Tatparam purushakhyateh guna vaitrishnyam.

Once you know the nature of your being - total bliss and total pleasure - even the fear about the *gunas* and the fear about the world will disappear. It is like diabetic patients being afraid of sweets. The sight of sweets frightens them because they are forbidden. But the one who has sweetness in him does not mind if there are sweets near them.

This is *parama vairagya* – supreme dispassion, ie., not being scared or running away from the world but being in it; completely centered.

People have very peculiar ideas about enlightenment. Every culture and religion has got its own ideas about it. In the Christian religion a rich man cannot be enlightened. It is impossible. You have to be poor to be enlightened. From the Christian point of view, Rama could not be enlightened. He was a King. How could a King be enlightened? Even if a camel could go through the eye of a needle, a rich man could not be enlightened.

Once, I was travelling from Bangalore to Delhi. I met a gentleman at the airport. He was a Christian priest. He looked at me and smiled. I smiled back and he came over to talk to me. Addressing me as his dear brother, he said that he felt like talking to me. Being encouraged by me to do so, he said that I seemed to be a very nice person. Then, he asked me if I believed in Jesus. I replied that I did. He was a little stunned. He asked me again if I really believed in Jesus. When I reaffirmed that I did, he asked me if I wasn't a Hindu. I replied that perhaps I was. Then, he pointed out that I believed in Krishna. I said that I believed in Krishna, too. He asked me how Krishna could be God. He was a butter thief. He was married. How could somebody who stole butter and who was married be God? Continuing, the priest said that Krishna could not give me salvation and Jesus was the only way. He said that he was also a Hindu at one time but he had converted to Christianity later. He said that from the time that he had become a Christian everything had begun happening. Jesus was taking care of him. Then, the priest advised me to convert to Christianity, too. And he was so sincere in telling this and in trying to convert me!

Jains do not consider Krishna to be enlightened because he had started the war. Arjuna had decided to renounce the world and take *sanyas*. But Krishna had brainwashed him and had made him fight in the war. Since Krishna was responsible for the big war, how could he be enlightened? Then, again he had been stealing butter and had so many wives. It was impossible that he was enlightened.

Jains do not think that an enlightened person, a *sadhu*, should even wear clothes. They think that such persons should always be naked. One who is not so, is not enlightened. How will it be known whether they are free from lust or not? What will be the proof? Jain *sadhus* are nude and they are considered enlightened. This is their idea of enlightenment. They do not consider anybody who eats and enjoys two meals a day to be enlightened. If a saint eats chocolate, he is not considered a saint at all.

Buddhists have got their own method of determining who is enlightened and who is not. Somebody who sings, dances, and enjoys living in the world is not enlightened. Somebody who mingles with their family members is not enlightened. The enlightened have to renounce their family. I have seen many of these so-called *sanyasis*. They are so afraid of meeting their own family. They fear that they could develop attachment for them again.

I remember in one of the *ashrams*, an inmate, a so-called *sanyasi* and renunciate, would not meet his mother, an old lady who was nearly seventy year old, when she would go there to meet him. He would meet everybody else. What had this poor old lady done that he would not even meet her? She would cry. Many of the renunciates - the so-called nuns, brothers and fathers are very cruel to their own family people because that is their idea of renunciation. Why cannot the close relatives be loved when everybody else can be? Why can't you see them with the same eye? This is a concept. Many *sanyasis* go through this difficulty about their family members.

Amidst all concepts about enlightenment, we forget the essence – dispassion and being centered. Being centered despite everything and living in the world. It is the second essential principle in Yoga. *Abhyasa* and *vairagya*.

Three *gunas* come in cycles in our life – *sattva, rajas, tamas*. When *sattva* comes, there is alertness, knowledge, interest, joy and happiness. When *rajo guna* comes, there are more desires, feverishness, restlessness, sadness, etc. When *tamo guna* comes, there is delusion, attachment, lack of knowledge, lethargy, etc. These three phases come in life in cycles. But one who is centered will watch, witness and just move through them, very naturally and easily, without being averse to any.

What happens when there is aversion? You promote it. You stay with whatever you are averse to. You continue to crave for whatever it is that you want. You allow the craving to continue.

Therefore, moving through the *guna* without craving or aversion is a real skill. And that is Yoga. *Yoga karmasu kaushalam* – the skill in action is Yoga. The word Yoga means skill - skill to live your life, to manage your mind, to deal with your emotions, to be with people, to be in love and not let that love turn into hatred. In this world everyone loves but that love does not stay the same for long. Soon, it turns into hatred; sometimes almost immediately. But Yoga is that skill, that preservative, that maintains love as love all the time.

Chapter 3

SAMADHI

Question: Dear Guruji, is it possible to get stuck in achieving a mood of dispassion, turning one's attention to the separation between self and thoughts, emotions and sensory data, and is it possible to see more clearly who you are? But if a habit is developed of separating oneself from everything in an artificial way, you will lose spontaneity, attunement with nature and will not fully engage in life by giving it your one hundred percent. How do you walk this tightrope, and how do you know if you are too far on one side or the other? Thank you, Jai Guru Dev.

Guruji: Dispassion does not divide you. In fact, it connects you. It connects you to the present moment so totally that you can be one hundred percent in anything that you are doing. When you are not dispassionate, then what happens? You are linked to the past or the future. You are not one hundred percent connected to the present and are more divided. So when your mind is hoping for something in the future or regretting the past, it is not hundred percent with the moment – that means it is divided already.

When you are fully centered while doing anything in the world, then you are hundred percent with every moment. You may be eating, and you are eating hundred percent. You enjoy every bit of it. You can feel every sip of the soup you are having. Every bite of the food tastes great. Every sight is fresh and new. So your love is like the first love every moment. When you look at anybody or anything, they are all charming to the core; as if you are seeing for the first time.

Dispassion does not take away the joy from you. Dispassion gives the joy which nothing else can give. There is a verse in *Shankaracharya* that says, "*Kasya sukham na karoti viraagaha*." What pleasure can dispassion not give? It gives all the pleasures because you are so totally in the moment. It puts you hundred percent in the moment. Every moment is a peak experience.

The so-called dispassion in the world seems so dry. People who think they are very dispassionate are melancholy. They are sad. They run away from the world and then they call it dispassion. Then, they say that they have renounced the world. This is no renunciation or dispassion. People who escape because of failure, misery, sorrow, or apathy feel that they have dispassion. Dispassion is something more precious, more refined, and more valuable in life. If you are dispassionate, you are always centered - full of joy and contentment. Anybody would like to be like that.

There is a story about Diogenes of Greece. When Alexander the Great saw him, he was being carried out to be sold as a slave. The people who were taking him to be sold also looked like slaves. Diogenes announced that he was a slave and asked loudly who wanted to buy him. Because he was roaring like a lion, it was difficult for the people to make out who was the slave and who was selling the slave.

Before Alexander the Great came to India, people in his country had told him that if he found some *sanyasi* here he should bring them back with him; that, they were very precious and were there only in India. So, when he was in India he ordered that some *sanyasis* should come to him. But, nobody would come. He then sent a message threatening them. He said that if they did not come, he would chop off their heads. Even then, nobody came. So he said that he was going to take away their books – the four Vedas and some other scriptures, too. The pundits agreed and said that they would give him all their books the next day. Overnight, the pundits made their children memorize all the manuscripts. And then they gave them to Alexander. They told him that they did not need them any more. Alexander got the manuscripts but he wanted a *sanyasi*, and a *sanyasi* would not come. Finally, he had to go to one *sanyasi* and threaten him saying that he would chop off his head if he did not go with him. The *sanyasi* replied that Alexander could do so if he wanted. The mighty emperor could not even look into *sanyasi's* eyes. He could not stand the power of dispassion that he saw there. Here was a person who, for the first time, did not care for an emperor.

When Alexander was in India, some people presented him some golden bread in a plate. And he said that he was hungry and wanted some real bread. They replied that he was an emperor, and how could he eat mere wheat bread. So, they had prepared golden bread for him. Alexander said that they were making fun of him and he was starving and wanted real bread. Hearing this, the people got some real bread. They asked him whether such bread was not available in his country. And why had he conquered so many places? Was it to get bread and if he too ate the same bread that was eaten in India? This shook Alexander for a moment. He felt that it was the truth. What was the point in conquering country after country. All that he needed was to live peacefully and happily. When he did not have that happiness and peace, and when he did not have that care and concern for his people, putting his stamp on all the villages and towns had no meaning.

So it seems Alexander said that, when he died, his hands should be kept open. He wanted the people to know that, though he conquered so many countries, Alexander the Great was going with empty hands. That he could not take a thing from this earth.

Dispassion is the strength in you. Even if the Lord of the Wealth comes, you do not need to take anything from Him. That is the strength of dispassion. It is not arrogance. It is centeredness. If you are so centered and calm, then you can understand that everyone who has come to this world has come to give something and not to take anything from here. A very different shift takes place.

The next sutra is:

वितर्कविचारानन्दास्मितारूपानुगमात् सम्प्रज्ञातः

Vitarka vichaara aananda asmita roopa anugamat sampragyaatah.

What is the purpose of this *sadhana*? *Vitarka* - when your mind has a special logic to pursue in the world and to perceive the truth. *Tarka* means logic. *Kutarka* means wrong logic – when the intention is not right and the logic is applied only to find fault; when you know deep inside you that something is not right, but you still logically prove that it is right.

Vitarka is special logic. You may be talking about dispassion and logically you are understanding it, and this logical understanding, hearing or talking has a certain effect on your consciousness. It elevates your consciousness. You are in a different space. This is *samadhi*.

Samadhi means equanimity. "*Dhi*" is the intellect – the

faculty that sustains you; faculty of consciousness. Now, we are in a state of *Samadhi*, because we are talking about the Self with a definite logic, an undeceivable logic. Logic can always change. Mere logic can change. You can put it on one side or you can put it on the other. There is no loyalty. But *vitarka* is a logic which cannot be condemned, which cannot be reversed. For example, if somebody is dead then it is obvious that he is dead. You know that the life that was there in the body is not there anymore. And that is the end. At that moment, your consciousness is in a different state. When you are not emotionally connected to anybody, what is happening to your consciousness? You feel that it is the end, for instance, when a movie is over, there is a feeling that all is over. When people walk out of the movie theatre, they are in a particular state of consciousness. They come out of a musical concert with a feeling that it is over. It is the same for a festival or for a course. When a course is over, the participants say that it has ended and they leave. The show is over. At that moment, there is a definite logic followed in the mind - irrefutable logic, irreversible logic that triggers your consciousness. It is so obvious.

Life is like this. It is so obvious. Everything is changing. They are bound to change; to dissolve and disappear. This *vitarka* elevates one's consciousness. One does not have to sit with the eyes closed or eyes open. The feeling of "I," the consciousness is all that is. Everything is empty. Everything is in a state of fluidity. The whole world is just a quantum mechanical field. This is *vitarka*. The entire science is based on *tarka*, irrefutable *tarka* of it, the quantum physics or whatever you call it. That is *vitarka*. V*itarka anugama samadhi*. This is a *samadhi*.

Then comes *vichara*. *Vicharanugama*. In *vichara*, there are all the experiences – smell, sight, visions, taste or sounds. When you meditate, these are all called *vicahraanugama samadhi*; all experiences and thoughts - observing the thoughts that come and go. There are two states of mind that surface in you often. One is a thought which disturbs you and the other is a thought that does not disturb you, but that which just hovers around in your consciousness and you are aware of it. You are in *samadhi*; you are in an equanimous state of mind. At the same time, there are thoughts hovering. It is a part of meditation. Thoughts exist and experiences exist. This is a second type of *Samadhi,* or awareness.

The third is *anandaanugama – ananda* which means a blissful state. Have you noticed that after you do *Kriya*, you are in a different space? When you sing *bhajans,* you are in a different space of *samadhi*. The mind is still elevated. The consciousness is still elevated and equanimous but it is in ecstasy. The *samadhi* is ecstasy; is *anandaanugama samadhi*. This is also a meditative state. This is a meditative state in which you are in ecstasy, and then there is a meditative state in which you are with some experiences, some thoughts, some ideas or some fleeting feelings hovering around. There is a third such state in which you have an irrefutable and logical understanding of creation. So, there are three such states.

Now, the fourth state is *asmitaanugama samadhi*. This is really the deep experience of meditation, wherein you do not know anything. There is just the awareness that 'you are'. You just know 'you are' but you do not know who, what or where you are. Nothing else is known but the experience of 'I am' – *asmita* – 'I am present.' This is the fourth state of *Samadhi*, or meditative state.

All these four are called, *samprajyata*, which means that there is consciousness in all this. There is an outflow of awareness throughout.

Now, how do you achieve them?

The next sutra is very simple.

विरामप्रत्ययाभ्यासपूर्वः संस्कारशेषोऽन्यः

Viraama pratyaya abhyaasa poorva sanskaara shesho anyah.

By 'doing' something you cannot experience, you cannot achieve this awareness. You cannot bring up the intelligence and the alertness in you by effort. It can be done only without effort; with relaxation - by relaxing and reposing in the Self. *Viraama pratyaya* – resting. *Abhyaasa poorva* means the practice of resting - conscious relaxation and rest.

Unconscious rest is sleep which we are forced to do by the nature. You are not resting voluntarily; you are forced to. When you are very tired, it feels as if nature is pulling you down and forcing you to rest. You are not resting voluntarily. It is only in meditation that you really rest because you are consciously resting. You allow the rest. Otherwise, your rest swallows you. Sleep is putting yourself to rest and meditation is resting on your own. This is *abhyasa*. This is practice - practice of deep rest consciously. *Viraam aabhyaasa poorva*.

Then comes *samskara sheshonyaha*. For some people, this comes through old *samskaras*, impressions. Some people have to do a lot of practice in order to be calm and equanimous; in order to bring up more awareness in them. For some people it happens due to some old impressions of past-lives. Some people start opening up right from their birth or they do so at a particular period in their lives. *Samskara sheshonyaha*. Some people suddenly open up to some spiritual experience after they are thirty or forty years old. Then, they have more awareness. But unfortunately, most of these people get misguided. They get a little experience and then they go on with all kinds of prophecies about the end of the world, etc. They may have read about some prophecies somewhere in the Bible. Then, an experience becomes so real to them that they see visions. And they begin to make prophecies. This is because they have no knowledge of the root of Yoga. They may see a white light coming down, and they will exclaim that something would be happening. People get misled by such evangelic experiences. But, someone who knows the roots will be aware of all about such experiences.

We should know that they are all from *samskara shesha* - some *samskaras* from the past. That is a different type of *samadhi*.

भवप्रत्ययो विदेहप्रकृतिलयानाम्

Bhava pratyayo videha prakritilayaanaam.

This goes more into an esoteric line. *Samadhi* does not belong to just a particular level of existence. It surpasses that level, too. It goes into other worlds also. People who do not have a body can be affected by the meditation, too. When you meditate you are not just bringing harmony within yourself but you are influencing the subtle layers of creation and the subtle bodies at all the different levels of existences in the creation. So, your meditation influences those people who lived hundreds of years ago - their consciousness and their minds. It influences the minds and consciousness of people who would be living in the future, too. Though, life is there in every moment, it is also infinite. Your life has been here from centuries and will continue to be here for centuries more.

There are different types of *yogis*. One is called *videha*, means one who does not have a body. You can go on feeling as though you have no body, and the mind will be in a high state of equanimity. And those who do not have a body also come within the influence and effect of Yoga. It is the same with *Prakriti laya*. *Prakritilaya* means those who are completely submerged in nature. They also attain the same state of equanimity. They are so away from the material existence that they are not even aware of it. *Videha* is complete unawareness of the body and surroundings. Your eyes are closed and you are totally immersed. Then, too are you in *samadhi*, in a state of meditation. When you are looking at a mountain or at a sunset, *Prakritilaya* is taking place in you. You are merging with nature at that moment.

You are looking at the sunset. The sun is setting. You are there along with the sun and the vision that you are having about it. And then in a while you are not aware of yourself. You are just aware of the sun. When you are watching a mountain, sometimes you forget yourself. You have no awareness of your thoughts, mind or body. No awareness at all. This is *Prakritilaya samadhi*.

However, when this happens, your mind suddenly pops up with the thought that you are being stupid just staring away at water. You think that you should better use your time and do something else. You may think of somebody or something. Then you are not dissolving in nature.

Prakruti laya is a big practice. People sit in solitude for years till all thoughts disappear. And all that they are left with is emptiness. You can try doing this as an experiment when you are very worried or tensed. Just sit by a flowing river or stream and keep looking at the water. Within a few moments, you feel as though there is a magnetic pull; that your mind is being pulled in the direction of the current. Then, sit on the other bank and do the same thing. Then you'll see that your mind is being pulled in the other direction. That is why many people who want to jump into a river and commit suicide, cannot do so once they look at the flowing water. Something happens in them at the sight of flowing water. There is a shift, and they can no longer commit suicide. This happens because, by looking at the water, there is a change in the vibrations of their mind, the *prana* in the system. In a short while, all their anguish, delusions and whatever was tormenting them flows away. They become fresh. People love the ocean because there is more *prana* there; more ozone. And when you go on looking at the waves and waves and waves and waves, it washes something off. This is *Prakritilaya* meditation, where you are dissolving yourself with nature.

And *videha* means knowing that you are not the body; that you 'have' a body and the body is yours. But that you are not the body. This is *videha*. This sutra has been so wrongly interpreted over the centuries. People have wrongly understood it again and again.

Patanjali said that these things will suit certain people at certain times. It is not a practice which is done everyday by everybody. For instance, all the people do not go into the mountains every day. It is done by certain people at certain times. This leads to *samadhi*.

Then comes,

श्रद्धावीर्यस्मृतिसमाधिप्रज्ञापूर्वक इतरेषाम्

Shraddha veerya smriti samaadhi pragyaapoorvaka itareshaam.

This is the most vital sutra.

Shraddha means faith. Faith creates such good qualities in your consciousness. It is made stable, steady and solid. Doubt in consciousness makes you very vulnerable, fearful, uncertain - fluid. But faith makes you solid. Faith brings totality in you. It pulls together all the loose ends of your consciousness. It integrates your whole personality. Doubt scatters and destroys you. It disseminates you and your energy. It pulls you apart. Dissemination of energy is doubt. Consolidation of your energy is faith. The feeling when you have faith is a form of consolidation; a strength. That is why Jesus also said faith is your strength. They are synonymous - faith and strength. When you are strong and bold, you have faith. When you are weak and feeble, you have doubts. Doubt and uncertainty are signs of weakness. Faith is strength. When there is faith, then *samadhi* is also achieved. And there is equanimity. Meditation takes place just out of faith.

And then there is *veerya*. *Veerya* is one hundred percent vigour or force, courage and vitality. It is total courage and valour; the valour with which a country is defended by its army. What happens here is that all the energy in the system comes together. We fight for our country when it is in danger; when the religion is in danger. This is how the valour rises in people. It is not done without any joy. In that moment of valour and extreme sense of patriotism, there is tremendous joy. That is why this world has wars again and again. If people completely condemn wars and if nobody likes them, then they cannot take place. Though the after-effects of war are very unpleasant, its course is very thrilling. People enjoy thrilling movies for the same reason. A thrill is a sense of *virya*, valour.

Every cell in our body becomes united and the whole consciousness becomes one. The defence system gets awakened in you. This is strength. When the defence system peaks, it is very joyful because there is equanimity, too. There is a sense of patriotism, devotion and gratitude. That sense of patriotism, or valour, or vigour also takes you into a state of meditation.

Shraddha veerya smriti. Smriti means memory. Once you have had a very peaceful and beautiful state of mind, the very memory of an experience will make you re-live that experience. Memory of *samadhi* reproduces memory of one's being; of the Self, freedom, devotion, surrender, love and joy. This takes you back to your Self. Often, we do not remember nice things. What we keep remembering are negative things. We do not remember compliments but we remember insults.

Yoga is turning the wheel around to remember those wonderful moments you have had. Sit and be with it, and with that very memory your entire being gets back to that wonderful state.

Smriti samadhi prajnapoorvaka. Then awareness is gained through *samadhi*, deep meditation, equanimous mind, and the result is *samadhi, prajna.* Equanimous mind gives rise to a heightened awareness.

So, these are the avenues and ways by which you can blossom in life.

These are the ways of being aware of the Self, and the next sutra is

तीव्रसंवेगानामासन्नः

Teevra samvegaanaam aasannah.

Often we give third, fourth or fifth preference to our practices. First preference is always given to worldly things - our survival, and last preference to anything that is spiritual. Then the spiritual growth will be slow.

Patanjali said, "*Teevra samvegaanaam asannaha.*"

When you give first preference to your spiritual practices, then it is easier. The focus of your life should be spiritual growth and peace. Then, all the other things will be around it.

Your first and foremost commitment in life is to be with Truth, and to evolve in Truth. This should be followed by your duties and responsibilities, social obligations, etc. If this is followed it is very easy for you to become aware of your self.

Teevra samvegaanaam asannaha. It is very easy for one who gives it first preference; one whose mind really wants to be aware.

Even then, there are three levels of commitment.

मृदुमध्याधिमात्रत्वात्ततोऽपि विशेषः

Mridu madhyaadhimantratva tatoh api visheshah.

Mridu can mean the rate: slow, medium or fast.

There are also three grades of people –the first are those who are one hundred percent into spiritual practices, then there are those who are not completely into it, and the last category are those who do the practices because they have to do it.

Then the next sutra says

ईश्वरप्रणिधानाद्वा

Iswara pranidhaan dwa.

Just by devotion to God, one-pointed devotion to God also *samadhi* is possible.

Chapter 4

WHO IS GOD

Surrendering to the Lord, you can achieve the fully blossomed state of consciousness. Now, what is the Lord? Who is the Lord? Where is He? It is easy to say surrender to God, but what is God? Where is God? Nobody has ever seen God. What is it that rules this world?

You will find that it is love that rules the world. The centre core of the existence rules this whole universe. Just like the sun is the centre of the solar system and rules all the planets, love is the core of your life. Love is beyond your changing body, changing thoughts, and changing feelings. It is the very centre, core, of your existence, which is very subtle and delicate. It can be called love or anything else. That consciousness, the core of existence is responsible for this whole creation. There lies the Lordship. A bird feeds its young ones because of love. A flower blossoms because of love. Ducks hatch eggs because of love. Cows take care of their calves because of love. Kittens are taken care of by cats because of love. Have you seen how monkeys care for their young ones? Love is in-built in creation. This is how the creation is functioning.

That is why Jesus said, "Love is God. God is love." They are synonymous.

Patanjali analysed this very beautifully in the next sutra. What is that state of consciousness? Who is Lord? That consciousness is free from misery or suffering. What is suffering?

क्लेशकर्मविपाकाशयैरपरामृष्टः पुरुषविशेष ईश्वरः

Klesha karma vipaaka aashaya aparamrishtah purusha vishesha eeshwarah.

It indicates that core of consciousness which is free from suffering. There are five types of suffering.

One is ignorance, *avidya*. When your consciousness is filled with ignorance, then there is restlessness. There is unhappiness and suffering. Misery is due to ignorance. Ignorance is giving importance to something which is not important; that which is not worthy of that importance - thinking that something that is changing to be permanent, imagining something which is not joyful to be joyful, considering something impure to be pure, etc. Someone may have said something unpleasant to you. Those were just words that came out of his mouth and vanished. But, to regard them as permanent and brooding over them is ignorance. Someone's comment about you is a fleeting wave of thought or energy which came and went. He may not even have that opinion later. But you keep that ever in your mind as his opinion about you, which is not true. This is one example of ignorance. So, the consciousness needs to be devoid of ignorance and free from misery.

Asmita means "me" or "I." This feeling of "me, I" is the second cause of suffering. That is the reason we do the Hollow and Empty process. When we do it, there is no "I". You exist as though you are not there. You exist like a flower; like a cloud. You exist like the space – free, and hollow and empty, rather than as if you are somebody - "I, I, me, me." *Asmita* is feeling what people think about you, what you want from them, how you could take advantage of them, whether they consider you to be good or bad, etc. This gives you misery. Nothing else can give you misery – need give you misery. Your own idea of "me, mine, me, mine," not being one with the existence, having a separate feeling and identity, or having a superiority or inferiority complex give you misery. In fact, all those people who consider themselves intelligent and everybody else fools, know deep down that they are really the bigger fools. To avoid thinking of their foolishness, they consider everybody else crazy or foolish. This *asmita* eats you up, and is the cause of your sufferings.

Raaga – means a strong craving for anything and *Dwesha*, means aversion or hatred. And *abhinivesha*, fear. Craving, aversion, fear, "me, I" – that separate entity of "I" - and ignorance; these are the five sources of misery. The Lord is devoid of these five miseries. That consciousness deep down in you is devoid of them. You may be miserable or craving for something. But, if you really go to the core of your existence, you are free from it. Outwardly, you may be hating somebody, but in the core of your existence there is no hatred. There is fear only at the circumference; so also ignorance. At the core of your existence, there is no fear or ignorance. There is no 'you' there.

When these five *kleshas* are eliminated even at the circumference, then whatever is in the centre becomes very eminent. The Lordship in you blossoms and the God in you is manifested. God is that *purusha*, that being, or Lord, which is devoid of these five *kleshas*, sufferings or miseries and He is also devoid of karma.

There are four types of karmas. One is the karma, which will give merits. There is another type of karma - action which brings you demerits. You may do something good for somebody, and they feel good about it and may thank you for it. They thank from their heart, and that brings you a good karma. Then again, you may do something bad to somebody. And they suffer because of it and are miserable. That brings you karma of demerit. And there are certain karmas which have the combination of merit and demerit. This is the third type of karma. The fourth type of karma is devoid of both merit and demerit – for example, you go for a walk in the evening or you are vacuum-cleaning the hall. These actions have no merit or demerit. They are just actions. But if you are doing it for somebody, eg., you are helping someone in the kitchen, then that is an action of merit. If you are cutting the vegetables and cooking food for everybody, then it is an action of merit.

Actions which give merit, which give demerit, which give mixed results and which has no results at all (neutral results) are the four types of karmas. At the very core of your existence, the being is free from all these karmas. It has no karma. Whatever action that comes forth from the Lord is not attached to any karma.

Vipaaka is fruit of the action; consequences of the action. Enjoying or suffering the fruit of an action is not applicable here. This does not touch that core of your being and existence, which is the Lord of creation; that consciousness which is free from this.

And *Aashaya*. *Aashaya* means latent desires or impressions, opinions, seeds, etc. So when a consciousness or a being is free from *klesha*, misery, karma, *vipaaka* – the fruit of action, and *aashaya*, the impressions of actions, then that being or consciousness is *Eshwara* or Lord. And the Lord is not somewhere in the sky but in your heart. It is in every being's heart. Your actions and the events taking place around you do not touch the central point of your life. That central core remains a virgin. Jesus was born to a virgin. This means that Jesus, the Lord was born to this virgin area deep inside you which is untouched by any events or happenings in life.

Purusha vishesha – that special being is the Lord when your external mind is worshipping the core of your being. All worship is done by the mind to its Being. It is like the circumference collapsing into the centre. When a boundary collapses to the centre, what happens? The area, which had been enclosed by the circumference, becomes infinite; becomes limitless. When our little chattering mind prays, it does so to the Infinite Being that you are. That is prayer – when you ask your Lord to help you.

Krishna meant this when He said that one may pray to whoever he wants. But the prayer goes to only Him because he is the core of existence. You may worship one form of God. Another may worship a different form. A third person may worship yet another form. Essentially, worship is just an act of dissolution - a sugar doll or candy getting dissolved in water. It does not matter at which point it gets into the water. It is going to dissolve and merge. Just like this, worship dissolves the mind of the worshipper. It is the act of dissolving the mind into its being; the being which is free from *klesha, karma, aashaya* and *vipaaka*. This takes place almost instantaneously. That is why there is no difference between God, Guru and your Self.

Eshwaro gururatmeti murti bheda vibhagine.

It is just a matter of using different words which are synonymous. The Master is the core of your being. And so is the

Divine who rules this entire creation.

स पूर्वेषामपि गुरुः कालेनानवच्छेदात्

Sa poorveshaam api guruh kaalenaanavacchedaat.

This being, this consciousness is Guru. It is a guide to even the ones who were here before. This is because there is no break in time, as far as the consciousness is concerned. There is something similar in the Bible. God had said that He was Abraham before and had taught people who were before Him. The same thing is touched upon by Krishna when he told Arjuna that He had taught Ikshvaku and Manu. And Arjuna wondered how could Krishna have taught them? They had been born long ago and Krishna was his contemporary. So Arjuna exclaimed that he was terribly confused already. And that he should not be told those things - that Krishna was a Guru to people who were living thousands of years before Him. How could it be possible?

Then Krishna said that Arjuna did not really know Him. That He had come so many times to this world and Arjuna, too, had come many times. He had forgotten but Krishna knew it all. He had taught at that time and he was teaching then, too and would continue to teach in the future.

The Guru principle is the same because there is no break in time. It continues. Jesus is continuing throughout. It is not that he stopped somewhere. People may think that He will be coming in the future. *Poorveshamapi guruhu.* He was, is and will be the Master at all times because there is no break in time.

तत्र निरतिशयं सर्वज्ञत्वबीजम्

Tatra niratishayam sarvagyatvam beejam.

This indicates that the seed of all-knowing is in that state of consciousness. This is very important. *Tatra niratishayam sarvajna beejam.* The seed of all-knowing is present in a very subtle manner. At this point people get confused. They wonder that if Lord Krishna knew everything why did He try to pacify all concerned, and try to stop the war three times. He knew that a war was going to take place. But, He never told Arjuna this, and also that he was going to win this war. Instead, He told him that if Arjuna won the war, he would rule the world. And, if he lost it he would go to heaven. It did not seem as if He knew everything and, consequently, the result of the war. He did not give the right answers, the right knowledge or the right instructions. He did not indicate the future results. So if Krishna was Lord and knew it, why did he not reveal it? This is the second question that comes.

Tatra niratishayam sarvajna beejam. This seed of all-knowing is present. For example, you have a dictionary. You can check the meaning of any word that you want. But, you do not need to memorize every word there. Nor do you need to know all the words in the dictionary all the time. You may open yourself up to this highest form of your consciousness. At that moment, you have all knowledge - you can know and feel all the beings in the world. You can know how many are there and what they are doing - some may be waking up, some going to bed, some taking baths, some in their motorcars, some fighting, some eating and some doing other activities. This is just about the people.

But take into account the entire living creatures. There are so many connected activities - so many chickens are hatching, so many are being slaughtered; so many buffaloes are wandering around and so many cows are chewing the cud; so many monkeys are jumping from tree to tree. There are so many ants, cockroaches, flies, mosquitoes, amoebas, etc. There are and billions of viruses and bacteria. Many are dying, many are being born and many are hatching. Many are growing. There is an enormous activity going on at any moment. But, amidst this enormous activity you just wonder what a particular person is doing. This takes so much effort and is not worth it.

Sometimes, people ask me how I know their most well-kept secrets; those which they have not told anybody. I tell that I do not know how but that I know. And then sometimes, I search for my own keys which I have misplaced. This is more confusing to such people. They wonder how I know something that they have never told anybody but how I do not know where I have kept my keys! I tell them that it is possible - just like they do not know how many hair they have on their heads? They know they have hair, but they do not know how many.

So, knowledge and ignorance co-exist. Even if you pull one hair you are aware of it. That is why it is said, "*Tatra niratishayam sarvajna beejam.*" This seed of all-knowing is present in the consciousness. It is amazing that it is present there. *Tatra niratishayam* – The seed of all-knowing is present in the Lordship; in that state of consciousness,

Poorveshaamapi guruhu kaalenaanavacchedaat – This consciousness is the Master of even those who lived in this world earlier.

Tasya vaachakaha pranavaha – how do you address the consciousness? Patanjali said to address it as *OM*. It is the nearest sound that it could be addressed with because when *OM* is said, the *prana*, and the consciousness is total. *OM* is constituted of "Aaa", "Ooo" and "Mmm". When you say "Aaa", the prana is in the lower portion of the body; with "Ooo" it is the middle and with "mmm" it is in the top portion of the body. When you say, "*OM*," the *prana* is total; it is complete.

"*OM*" is the sound which is so special. It is the nearest sound that could be used to address this totality of consciousness. The "*OM's*" distorted form is Amen in Christianity and "Amen" or "*Ameen*" in Islam. That is why "*OM*" is the one sound which is accepted by all the religions in the world. All of them have an important word which is "OM", or very close to "OM". So "OM" is one sound which comes very close to this totality of consciousness. All other names are just on the periphery.

तज्जपस्तदर्थभावनम्

Tajjapastadartha bhaavanam.

This is another important sutra. If you say *Japa* loudly, the very sound can remind you of that state of feeling during *Japa*. For example, if you say mango, the word itself makes your mouth water. Immediately there is a reaction and there is a feeling. Saying "Christmas" immediately generates a feeling of celebration and giving and receiving gifts.

So, *tajjapastadartha bhaavanam* – means that when you say "OM," you remember that totality of your being - that being which is at the very core of this existence, that life which is free from misery and which is all unconditional love. The sound "OM" reminds you of the Lord of the Creation.

ततः प्रत्यक्चेतनाधिगमोऽप्यन्तरायाभावश्च

Tatah pratyak chetna adhigamo apyantaraayaabhaavascha.

When you reach the core of your existence and when there is a feeling of elevation, consciousness dawns in you. It is a different form of consciousness. Your mind gets totally transformed. There is clarity in your thinking and in your feelings. The whole body undergoes a transformation. You become alive and full of *prana* and all the obstacles get removed from your way. Just the memory of the Lordship, of the Divine can remove obstacles from your way.

There are nine obstacles:

व्याधिस्त्यानसंशयप्रमादालस्याविरतिभ्रान्तिदर्शनालब्ध भुमिकत्वानवस्थितत्वानि चित्तविक्षेपास्तेऽन्तरायाः

Vyaadi Styaana samshaya pramaada aalasya avirati bhrantidarshana aalabdha bhoomikatvaan avasthi tatvaani chitta vikshepaaha aste antaraayaah.

The first obstacle is *vyaadi*. It means illness in the body. Then comes *styaana*. It is illness of the mind – being mentally retarded and having an inability to comprehend, to listen, to understand, to follow, and to practice.

Many of you will become ill when you do a course. When you start doing some practice or meditation, you will have pains in various parts of your body. It is an obstruction or obstacle in the path of Yoga. If you are watching television, nothing happens, but if you sit for meditation, your body becomes restless and there are pains here and there.

The next obstacle is *samshay* or doubt. The mind is bogged down by doubts. There are three types of doubts. One is a doubt about oneself. You wonder if you are good enough. You feel that you cannot do something that is required to be done. You may see that everyone else is meditating and in a blissful state or that they are in a very happy and pleasant mood. You feel that it is just you who are suffering and that you are no good. You do not think that you can ever make it. So, initially there is a doubt about yourself. And then doubts arise about the techniques. You may feel that they may not do you any good and that you should try some other technique. Next, doubts about the teacher arise.

These three types of doubts can hamper progress. Your doubt is always about something that is good. You never doubt the negative. You always doubt the positive. You never doubt your depression. You never wonder if you are really depressed. But, you will certainly doubt your happiness. You will wonder if you are happy; if what is making you happy is really what you wanted. Doubt is the third obstruction.

Pramaada is the next obstacle. It means doing something wrong willfully; doing it with some motive. You may know that certain things are not good for you. Despite this, you continue to do it. Conversely, you may know the need to do something, and then you do not do it, for instance, you know very well that you have to pay the tax and you don't pay it. Suppose you are sick and should not eat ice-cream, etc or that you should not overeat, yet you do so. You may have some sugar problem and should not eat much sugar. Despite knowing this, you go on eating sweets or chocolates. So, being careless and not being alert and attentive is another obstacle. This is *pramaada*.

Who Is God | 69

And, then comes *Aalasya* or laziness. You may be very active but when it comes to doing *asanas*, postures, exercises or *pranayamas*, you are lazy and do not do them. And that laziness can spread to any aspect of your life. You may intentionally not do something. Then again, you may feel a heaviness or laziness come over you.

Avirati means being obsessed with sensual objects and not letting them go. You may be hungry and eat some food. But after your tummy is full, then there is no point in thinking about food the whole day. It is the same if you want to see a beautiful place. Once you see it, your want should subside. You should not go on thinking about seeing a beautiful place all the time. All the actions of the sense organs should be limited to some time. It should be over after that. But thinking about something and being feverish about it all the time is *avirati* or obsession. You eat and after eating you should not think about it. The same applies for sex. You have had sex and it is over. You do not carry sex in your head twenty-four hours. People see blue-movies day and night. Their head gets hot. The body is incapable of functioning and mind is obsessed with the thoughts of sex. Even old people have this problem. They are seventy, eighty, ninety years old, but they are thinking about sex.

Then that is *avirati*, non-detachment.

It is said that Mullah Nasseruddin celebrated his seventy-fifth birthday. Someone asked him what he thought about girlfriends. Mullah replied that he should not be asked that question because he had stopped thinking of girls three days back.

Incompletion of any sexual experience creates an *avirati*, attachment to that sense object, and lack of non-attachment to that sense object. *Avirati* is a big obstruction in the path of Yoga, for it does not allow you to get centered. It just pulls you down and keeps you from moving on.

Bhrantidarshana is hallucination. You imagine that you are somebody special. Suddenly you think that you are a superstar. This is a problem with many people. Many seekers practice something and they get some visions. They get caught up in that vision because that vision is neither completely false, nor completely true. It is a mixture of some truth, and some falsehood. So people try to hold on to it. Many cults have been formed because of this *bhrantidarshana*. They have never really understood the obstacles that can come up in the path of Yoga. This is called *Yoga Maya*. *Yoga Maya* is a vision that brings a message; an intuitive message. You may be meditating and you will get an intuition to open the door because somebody is waiting for you. And when you do that, you really find that person waiting outside. And you will get very excited. You will think that God had told you about it. And this will happen again and again. This is because you are not completely hollow and empty. There are residues or traces of your desires, hatreds, and fears. These ideas will come from the form in which you see God or your Guru or through someone else. And it will give you ideas which will make you suffer. This happened to one of our devotees. She had various visions and most of them happened. She had one vision which indicated that she should not take her husband to the doctor; that, he would be cured without a doctor. She was already apprehensive of going to a doctor and averse to allopathic medicine. And when she had her vision, she became quite determined not to go to a doctor. Then, her husband's blood sugar level shot up and he was not treated for it. This resulted in his losing his eyesight. The devotee became very angry, feeling that her inner voice had deceived her. This really happened because of a lack of proper understanding. Most of the factors were alright; there was no impurity in them. But then her own fears and cravings influenced her intuitive thoughts with unpleasant results. This is an obstruction. That is why we should not gallop on the horses of delusions – *bhrantidarshana*. Many people get trapped in it.

Alabda bhoomigatva is the non-attainment of any state or *samadhi*, any peace, or tranquillity.

Sometimes, people feel that they have been doing various practices for many years but do not seem to be getting anywhere. They feel that they are just sitting and nothing happens. Just thoughts come and they have not attained any state. Non-attainment of any state or *samadhi*, any peace, or any tranquillity is another obstruction - the eighth obstruction. This is where one feels completely stuck and thinks that they are getting nowhere. But, despite these thoughts, they do not give up the practice. However, they feel stuck without any progress.

Then, comes *anavastitatva* which means instability. You may get some good experiences. You may feel very calm and wonderful. But the feeling does not linger. It evaporates quickly. This is another complaint.

These obstructions and obstacles cause *dukha*, sorrow. *Dourmanasya* means bitterness in the mind. *Dukha* or sadness gives way to bitterness, *dourmanasya*. You do not feel good with anybody. There is bitterness with others and there is bitterness with oneself.

Angamejayatva comes next. It means that your body is not obeying you; just like a drunkard. A drunkard wants to go to the left but his body takes him to the right. He wants to walk straight, but his body goes haywire. He tries to hold his glass but goes on putting his hand on the table away from the glass. This lack of coordination between the body and the mind is *Angamejayatva*. The body does not listen to you. You want to walk but the body does not move.

दुःखदौर्मनस्याङ्गमेजयत्वश्वासप्रश्वासा विक्षेपसहभुवः

Duhkha dourmanasyaangam ajayatva shwaasa prashwaasa

vikskepa sahabhuvah.

These are the five signs of the obstacles overtaking you - *Dukha* – sadness, *dourmanasya* – bitterness, *bhrantidarshana* – hallucination, *angamejayatva* – lack of co-ordination of the body; it is not listening to you, *shwaasa prashwaasa* - irregular, shaky and uncomfortable breathing. These are the *vikshepas* that come along with these obstructions.

The next chapter will deal with methods to get rid of them.

Chapter 5

OVERCOMING OBSTACLES

We have considered the nine possible obstacles in the path of Yoga. There is no tenth obstacle. Every possible obstacle has been included in these nine categories.

Patanjali was a scientist. In just a few words, he had said all that was to be said; that needed to be said. Along with these nine obstacles, the five indications, or signs of a disturbed mind are mentioned. That is *dukha* – sadness, *dourmanasya* – bitterness, *angamejayatva* – restlessness in the body, or lack of co-ordination in the body, *bhrantidarshan*-hallucination and irregular breathing - imbalance of your incoming and outgoing breath.

When you are happy, or excited, the incoming breath is longer and you are more aware of it. It is more prominent. If you observe the incoming and outgoing breath, you will note that there is a total imbalance. There is a big sigh, when you are unhappy, indicating heaviness and sadness. When you are joyful, you are just aware of your incoming breath. You are not even aware when you are breathing out.

These are the five signs, or side-effects, along with the obstacles. Now, how do you get rid of these obstacles?

The next sutra is - *eka tattva abhyasaha, tat pratishedhaartham eka tattva abhyasaha.*

To get rid of them, just go on doing one thing! When you just keep doing one thing, you will begin to get bored and restless. And the restlessness and boredom will take you to a peak that will bring clarity. This is the only way out. Our mind is troubled because it is dwelling on duality. It has choices before it and so is more confused. It wonders if it should do this thing or the other. And then it is jumping all around the place, and the mind is further divided. A divided mind causes misery and a one-pointed mind causes joy. At all those moments when you had been very happy, the mind had become one; had become whole. You had experienced joy, peace and bliss. Then, you had experienced life totally.

Duality, or divided mind, is the cause of fear and misery. So, if you keep doing two things or too many things, it is not *eka tattvaabhyaasa.* It is not one practice. So what is the *eka tattva*? It is attending to one principle. This one principle could be God, could be a matter, could be Guru or could be Self. It could be anything but you need to practice just one of those things - *eka tattva abhyasa.* Then, you get over all the other obstacles. All the nine obstacles can be got rid of. You can attend to one principle, only if there is certain amount of calmness and subtleness in the mind. Otherwise, even that does not seem to be possible.

In one-pointedness there is a certain degree of calmness in the mind. You see that one principle in everybody. You feel that you are present everywhere; that your Master is present everywhere. There is nobody other than your Master. He is everything for you or God is everything for you. Really, it is all you. There is nothing other than you. This is the skill in life - holding on to one principle and seeing that principle in everything. Our life has to be lived in the realm of multiplicity. In the world you live with many people and everybody is not the same. But how can you see the same thing in everybody? Nothing appears to be the same. No two people appear to be the same. But we need to see one thing in everyone. Look at and focus on that one principle. How is it possible?

Then Patanjali said that he would reveal another sutra.

The next sutra says,

मैत्रीकरुणामुदितोपेक्षाणां सुखदुःखपुन्यापुन्यविषयाणां भावनातश्चित्तप्रसादनम्

Maitri karunaa mudito upekshanaam sukha dukha punya apunya vishayaanaam bhaavanaatah chitta prasaadanam.

Patanjali said that there can be only four types of people in the world - people who are happy, those who are unhappy, those engaged in good and meritorious acts, and those engaged in bad and demonic acts. Happy people, unhappy people, meritorious and blessed people and sinful people– the four categories. And how do you deal with them?

Patanjali said to have *maitri* – friendliness with all those who are happy. If you do not, you will be jealous. You are jealous of people who are happier than you. But if you feel that you own them and that they belong to you, it does not bother you when they are very happy. You are never jealous about the happiness of someone very close and dear to you. The jealousy arises when the happy person is not connected to you totally. So, Patanjali said that you should be friendly with them.

You can see the same Self in everybody but the feelings will not be the same. It can differ for a beginner. You do not feel identified with everybody, though intellectually you may feel that it is only you who is in the other person; but your feelings still have their preferences since they are not fully cultured and established in the Self. Then, what preference will you have? Be friendly with those who are happy. If you are friendly with unhappy people, you too become unhappy. So Patanjali said that we should not be friendly with unhappy people. But we should be compassionate to them.

The second *bhava* which Patanjali has given is *karuna*. Have sympathy and compassion for people who are suffering. But do not be friendly with them because this friendship will drag you down and make you unhappy, too. If you are unhappy and they are also unhappy, then you will be able to help them. You may think that you should share the unhappiness of your friend. But then, you will not be able to share your happiness with them. So, you should not be friendly with unhappy people, but should be compassionate to them. There is a difference here. Be compassionate to them. *Karuna* is compassion. We do not know how to deal with people who are suffering. We make their beliefs stronger that God has been unjust with them, and that Nature has been so unkind to them. We agree with them that they are suffering. Saying this, we push them lower down the drain. Actually, we have been trying to pull them out. Instead, we do the opposite. We do this unconsciously. We should not pity people who are suffering. There is much difference between pity and compassion. When we pity, we are not pulling a person up. We are pushing them further down. Most of the people do this. With their pity, they make the belief of the suffering person more concrete about his sorrow in whatever limited logic of relative existence. If someone thinks that a great injustice has been done to them and they are miserable and on a self-pitying trip, we do not help them in any way if we pity them. They will have a confirmation that they are suffering. We will not help them in any way to wake up to the truth. We should have compassion for people who are suffering but not friendliness.

And we should be happy with people who are doing good

job, who are meritorious, who have lots of merit and who are blessed. We should become one with them; feel that we are doing the good job with them. Then, the sense of competition disappears and jealousy subsides. The tendency to find fault with people who are doing good things will disappear. People have a tendency to find faults if someone is good and blessed or is meritorious and doing some good work. At least they have done whatever they have done! The persons, who complain, normally, would not have done much themselves. Criticism comes from people who do not work. They just criticize others. We should not find fault with people who are doing some good work. We should feel happy about it. Do not find fault, but feel happy for those people who are doing good work. You do this when you will become one with them. If the right hand is doing good job, the left hand will appreciate it and will not stop the right hand from doing it. So it feels that it is a part of the other hand. It can hold the table and the paper, so that the other hand can hold the pen and write well. So, we should feel that those who are doing something good are a part of us, and that we are doing a good job along with them. We should feel happy about it. *Mudita* means happiness about people who are doing wonderful job. Share the happiness, feel happy.

Ignore those people who are committing sins. *Upeksha* – just ignore them in your mind. If somebody says something which is not true, just brush it off. It is not even worth thinking about.

But we do the reverse. We do not think of people who are doing meritorious work. But we keep on thinking about people who do sinful things and we don't just ignore them. All the newspapers will report about somebody who committed a murder or some other heinous crime. The story and the snaps of the criminals will appear in the papers.

Fortunately, of late there are some reports on the good and positive things happening to people. But this is comparatively very little. So, when you see people doing sinful things, you should educate them and then ignore them. You educate out of compassion and then ignore. Otherwise, you will think about their actions and get bothered. You may think somebody is imperfect. If you go on thinking this, then you will become imperfect. Then, you will be just as they are, maybe, even worse. Secondly, you are thinking that the person is wrong and you think you are right. If you look honestly at yourself, you will realize that you may be committing more crimes. If you point an accusing finger at somebody, then there are three fingers always pointing towards you. So, it is one is to three. You have three times more responsibility. But, if you stop differentiating between yourself and others, then you can just turn inward.

मैत्रीकरुणामुदितोपेक्षाणां सुखदुःखपुन्यापुन्यविषयाणां भावनातश्चित्तप्रसादनम्

Maitri karunaa mudito upekshaanaam sukha dukha punya apunya vishayaanaam bhaavanaatah chitta prasaadanam.

Patanjali knew the human mind very well. And he knew all the crooks and bumps in it. He knew that it could not have the same feeling towards everybody all the time. Feelings can be developed and they keep changing, too. So he said that we should have feelings of friendliness, compassion, joy, happiness, etc. and ignore or have *upeksha* – indifference for the sinful things. If this is done, our *chitta,* our mind would be pleasant. *Chitta prasaadanam* – it will become graceful, gracious. In that gracious and graceful mind, one-pointedness becomes easy. We should practice devotion to one thing or one aspect.

Then, Patanjali said that if all this was difficult, then he would give one more sutra!

प्रच्छर्दनविधारणाभ्यां वा प्राणस्य

Prachchhardana vidhaaranaabhyaam vaa praanasya.

Prachchhardana vidaaranaabhyaam - Breaking the natural rhythms of the breath, holding it and sustaining it in different rhythms. Patanjali has not mentioned *Sudarshana Kriya* directly. But in this sentence, there is a clue. You can trace our practices to that one sutra because we are doing the same thing here. We are not just breathing anyway we like. We are consciously breathing in a definite rhythm. That is *prachchhardana* - splitting. We are splitting the breath, dividing them and holding them with different rhythms. That is *Prachchhardana vidaaranaabhyaam vaa praanasya*. We are modulating the *prana* and the breath.

This also makes our mind focused.

Now, another sutra is

विषयवती वा प्रवृत्तिरूत्पन्ना मनसः स्थितिनिबन्धनी

Vishayavati vaa pravrittih utpannaa manasah sthiti nibandhani.

Suppose, it does not work and you feel it is not complete. Then *vishayavati*. This means that the mind can be stilled through any one object of senses. What happens in eye-gazing? You are looking at somebody for a few minutes. You gaze at that person from the bottom of your heart. At that time, your mind is not running here and there. You sit with your eyes closed. The mind is completely settled. We may sit for a meditation after singing *bhajans*. The mind has come to a standstill.

विशोका वा ज्योतिष्मती

Vishokaa vaa jyotishmati. The next sutra,

If you are, even for a few moments, with a person who is very unhappy and sad then you also start feeling depressed. And, if you are with someone who is very joyful and is bubbling with joy and enthusiasm, then you start feeling joyful, too. You have trained your mind to be happy or unhappy. If you have acquired the habit of being unhappy, then it becomes your second nature. You feel at home having a long face all the time. You would see this in the senior citizen homes. The very old people there have the habit of complaining. They just go on complaining, even when there is nothing to complain about. And they keep a long face and ever remain sad. You may have wondered why a person who is aged cannot be happy. They have done everything that they needed to do and wanted to do and they have everything that they need. But, they continue to be sad and depressed. Many people are unhappy because they are unable to work. Well, that is the body's nature. When one is eighty years old, and if he is unhappy because he cannot run as long as he could do when he was a thirty years old, then it is ignorance and foolishness. The other day, an elderly person, a senior citizen came to see me. I asked him how he was doing and if he was happy. He said that he had been able to run so many kilometres a day when he was younger and could do so much work. He could work sixteen hours a day. He said that, currently, he was unhappy because he could not work so much. He had begun to get tired after working for just four hours. He had begun to get tired after walking just one kilometre. Then, he asked me how he could regain his strength so that he could walk four miles a day. I asked him why he needed to walk four kilometers a day!

This happens because a person feels that he needs to be fit but his body will not obey. The mind thinks that he should be working because he had been working earlier. It wonders how come the person is not working, that he is growing old. This idea of growing old makes a person very unhappy. Nobody can get rid of this unhappiness for them because it is self-imposed. And with that unhappiness the person gets jittery, angry and tense. They get all the other negativities. They get soaked in them and die in that condition.

Patanjali gives this, *vishokaa*. *Vishokaa* means getting rid of the unhappiness. Feeling sad is just your habit. If you look into your mind and see that the sadness is simply unfounded and self-generated, it will disappear and you will become free from it. It is just a concept like the concept that people do not respect you. It is baseless. You may feel that you are not smart enough; that nobody cares for you. Why should you think so? Then, again you may feel that you are stupid. You are not so. Stupidity is only a comparative term. You may be considered wise by somebody who stupider than you. There is a scale for stupidity. There will certainly be people who are stupider than you. All these self-imposed ideas make you very unhappy. Look down the scale and you will feel that you are wise. Your comparisons can disturb you and make you sad. Do not compare yourself with anybody. You should feel that you can be happier. *Vishoka* – make your mind free of sadness which comes out of you concepts.

ज्योतिष्मती प्रज्ञा ज्योतिष्मती प्रज्ञा

Jyothishmati pragya, Jyothishmati pragya.

Consider your mind as a light, as a flame. Your consciousness is a flame. Your mind is a flame. You may forget this. Your entire body is functioning because of the presence of the mind as a flame in you. Otherwise, you will be like an unlit candle. What is a flame? How does a flame work? A flame burns because of oxygen. There is a combination of matter and oxygen and a flame comes into being.

What is life? Life is also the same. It uses oxygen and lives on some matter. Just as a flame lives on the wax, the wick and oxygen, your life and the mind uses the body and the food in the body as wax. The air is like the oxygen and exhibits activities in the body just as the flame exhibits its activity. The consciousness exhibits life. Life and light are very similar. If you put a bottle over a burning candle, it will be extinguished in a few moments. Similarly, if you are shut in a room, without any windows, you can live only for a few hours because you will not get enough oxygen. It is very similar. If you do whatever you do to the candle to your body, too, there will be the same reaction. If you put more wax into the candle, it will burn for a longer period. Similarly, if you put food into your body, then it will live longer. If the wick is burnt out, no amount of wax will make the candle burn. The wick has its own limitation. Similarly, no amount of food will sustain the body after some years of life. The body functions just like a wick. This body is holding on to the *jyotishmati pragya*.

Vishoka vaa jyothismati – get rid of unhappiness and be happy. At the same time know that your mind is made up of light. It is not matter. Your mind is energy, you are energy. *Jyotishmati.*

Next sutra is

वीतरागविषयं वा चित्तम्

Veetaraaga vishayam vaa chittam.

Keep your mind engaged in the thoughts of the Enlightened. Your mind is like water. Your mind is like water because, just as water assumes the shape of its container, your mind becomes like the thought you engage in. It develops all the qualities of whatever you put into it, namely, your thoughts.

So, in the next sutra Patanjali says *veetaraaga vishayam vaa chittam. Veetaraaga* is one. If you think of a calm person, then your mind also begins to assume his qualities. It starts feeling that peace and that quietness. This is because mind is like air. It is energy and is all pervading. Air does not have a location. It is not just fixed anywhere. *Veetaraaga Chitta* - Mind is all permeating. So it enters your system because it is also like ether. Your consciousness is ether and is all pervading.

Veetaraaga vishayam vaa chittam. But then you apply *raaga* and *dwesha* even here. That is why it is said that a Guru, or an enlightened person does not see one who is liberated from and is beyond cravings as a human being; as a person with likes and dislikes. Instead, they are seen as pure consciousness. *Veetaraaga vishayam vaa chittam,* as peace, as joy. Then, these radiances start. But, even if any thoughts come or likes and dislikes arise, we should not struggle with them, thinking that we should not have such thoughts. We should just let go and relax. *Veetaraaga vishayam vaa chittam.* It is very simple. When you do this, then immediately you will draw on that energy and will assume that form. You should try this on your own, you should experiment. Just think of somebody who is very nasty and you will begin to feel nasty emotions inside. If you think of somebody who is very jealous of you, then you will feel uncomfortable sensations. If you think of somebody who is into drugs and alcohol and who is very miserable, then you will feel all these knots coming up in your body and in your system. Think of somebody whom you love very much, and you will have nice feelings and sensations arise in you.

So *veetaraaga vishayam vaa chittam* – If you think of the enlightened, your consciousness becomes more and more alive and filled with light. That is why Jesus had said that if anybody had to go to His father, he had to go through Him; that there was no other way.

You have to be enlightened through the Master, because the Master is liberated. To be enlightened, you have to pass through your mind; go through your mind. And what can help your mind? The doorway with those vibrations and sensations. And these vibrations and sensations manifest in that body where the *chitta* is *veetaraaga* - is blossoming fully or is fully blossomed, without any hindrances. *Veetaraaga vishayam vaa chittam.*

Then comes

स्वप्ननिद्राज्ञानालम्बनं वा

Swapna nidra gyana aalambanam vaa.

It means the knowledge of sleep and dreams. This is very interesting. You sleep all your life but have never met your sleep. This is the irony. It is like a person who had lived all his life having millions with him but who did not know how to spend them and lived in poverty. It is like a person who is sitting at a dining table with a very delicious meal but who does not know that it is a meal. He does not know how to eat it and he is starving to death. The same is true with our life, too. There is sleep here but we do not know what it is. We dream every day and we have not known what dreams are.

What happens when you sleep? You let go of everything. If you hold on to even one thing, you cannot sleep. In sleep all your identity disappears. You are neither a male, nor a female. There is no male sleep or a female sleep. There is no rich man's sleep or a poor man's sleep. There is no intelligent person's sleep or a stupid man's sleep. Sleep is just sleep. In sleep you let go of all your identity; of all your likes and dislikes. You cannot carry anybody into your sleep. However dear somebody is, you cannot take them with you in your sleep. In your sleep, you are devoid of all your identity, your cravings, your aversions, etc. You let go of them all and just rest. You do not do anything.

This is exactly what meditation is – when you do not do anything. In meditation you do not do anything even for God or for yourself. You just let go of everything as you do when you sleep. The knowledge of sleep leads you to *samadhi*.

Ignorant people make dream a reality and enlightened people see this reality as a dream. Trying to interpret dreams is utter ignorance. Enlightenment is to realize this reality itself is a dream. If you tell an enlightened person about your dreams, he will tell you to forget about them and to wake up. However, somebody who does "dream interpretation" will give you various meanings for your dreams. They will put more ideas in your head, trying to interpret all the dreams. This is ignorance.

There are five types of dreams. The first are those that are fulfilment of your cravings and your unfulfilled desires. You may want to have an ice-cream or a pizza but you postpone it. Then, when you are asleep you have a dream in which you are eating a pizza or having a big scoop of ice-cream. You may have wanted to go for a walk with somebody and you could not do it. And then you dream that you are on such a walk. Your latent desires come up in dreams. Desires and fears are seen in dreams.

The second type of dream is when there is some stress released from the past. Past experiences are seen in such dreams.

The third type is an intuitive dream. It might be about what might happen in the future – an intuition.

The fourth type of dream is a combination of all the three – fulfilment, stress-release and intuitive.

And the fifth type of dream has nothing to do with you. It is about the place where you are sleeping. You may be in a hotel in Italy and you dream of the unfamiliar Italian language, and all the unfamiliar sounds that you have been hearing in that country.

So, these five types of dreams can occur. And you may not be able to categorize you dreams. Usually, it will be the fourth type, which is a combination of all five. Therefore, a wise person will just brush them aside. He will consider a dream to just be that, and nothing more. Even the reality of wakefulness is a dream. You may be in a place on one day and in another the next and in a third the day after. Your presence in a place in the past will seem like a dream. Similarly, what you are planning to do next week is like a dream right now. Your mind is more in a dream than in wakefulness.

There are only two states of consciousness. One is deep sleep or dream - day-dream or night-dream. Day dream - building castles in the air. This day-dreaming goes on and on in the mind, all the time.

But, once you know that you are day-dreaming, there is a gush of energy in you. You become alert. This alertness wakes you up to the reality. You are awakened. This awakening is *pragya*. It is *samadhi*. Only at that moment are you fully alive. Only then are you awake to the truth of what is. The rest of the time, you are sleep. You wake up even when you know that you have been in a deep sleep and have been dreaming.

And Patanjali has done a marvelous thing just quoting this one sutra. Knowledge of sleep awakens you. This is because when a person is asleep, he is not at all aware of it. The moment he knows that he is sleeping, he is already awake. A person, who is day-dreaming does not know it. And the moment he knows that he is day-dreaming, he wakes up to reality at that very moment, instantly.

When you are doing *Kriya* and *pranayam* and nothing is happening to you, you begin to day-dream or sleep. There can be only two possibilities. If you are day-dreaming, the *pranayam* cannot help you. It is very difficult for politicians to get into any *sadhana* because their mind is in a constant state of day-dreams. And the tragedy is that they do not know it. Their dreams are worth nothing.

Swapna nidra jnana aalambanam vaa. The knowledge of dream and sleep can also awaken you to the truth.

Next Patanjali said - *Yathaabhimmata dhyaanadhwaa.*

There are many different methods of meditations. You can be awakened by any one of methods. You can choose the one that suits you but you need to stick to it. You should not change it at all. If you take one path, you should go only on that path.

And, you should not change Masters at all. Otherwise, you will get very confused and messed up. All the ways are good. Take up one and just go deep into it, without criticizing the others. Then, you will be building it up in you.

यथाभिमतध्यानाद्वा

Yatha abhimat dhyaanadwaa.

There are different methods of meditation.

What is the sign of progress in this?

Patanjali said

परमाणुपरममहत्त्वान्तोऽस्य वशीकार:

Paramaanu parama mahttva antosya vasheekaarah.

Within the purview of your operation or life will come the smaller than the smallest to the bigger than the biggest. The nature will love you and start supporting you.

Chapter 6

STEADINESS IN SAMADHI

When the earth shakes for a few seconds, there is much disaster. You can exist on this planet because it is steady. Once in a while, it shakes and this throws the inhabitants off balance. A few seconds of this is enough to bring life to a standstill for many days.

There are natural calamities – flood, torrential rain, scorching heat. This disturbs life. You can be at peace only when the nature is at peace and is steady. At one time a couple of years ago there was snow fall in the Sahara desert in the middle of summer. In the same year, England was extremely hot during the winter months. This had never happened before.

Nature trembles once in a while. But your senses are trembling every day. When the senses are shaky, it is unable to behold, or hold the Lord within. This disturbs the peace in you. Like nature, there is peace only when the senses are steady. Meditation can happen when there is harmony in nature and in your senses. Your vision needs to be fixed. If not, then the mind is not in a meditative state. You should observe this when you sit for meditation. Are your eyes steady? Is your breath steady?

Is the *prana* haphazard or is it smooth and normal? When the senses are steady, the soul becomes peaceful. Your being and your spirit become steady. Your senses are shaken when they feel the joy which is the nature of Self in the objects that are outside. The senses can be considered to be a bridge. On one side are the objects that give pleasure, and on the other side is the Self. When the senses feel that more pleasure will come from the objects, they shake. Even when the senses shake for a few minutes, they become tired. Then, they are unable to enjoy or perceive the joy or experience it.

Recently, I had been to a blind school in India. There were one hundred and seventy-five children who were blind. They sang *bhajans* for half an hour. It was amazing the way they were singing the *bhajans* with all their heart. Our devotees felt that they had never experienced a *bhajan* session like that. The effect was so powerful. This was because they had sung with no distraction of sight. They did not look around while they were singing because they could not see. It was as if they were singing from a very deep, meditative state. Their whole being was in the *bhajans*.

These eyes which you think guide you and bring you light, bring you darkness too. This is because these eyes bring you all sorts of temptations - imagining that something is more beautiful than the other. The mind would be far more peaceful without the eyes. The eyes are the greatest distraction for the steadiness in the Self. Evil does not tempt you. Your eyes are good enough to do so. Someone had prayed to God not to give him any temptations and that he would find his own. The eyes find their own temptation.

This is the same with the ears. Sometimes, people switch on the radio and every few minutes change the station. They go on tuning to different stations. I knew one such person. He would not let anybody listen to one song completely or one program fully. After listening to a station for a few seconds, he would wonder what program would be on in another station. Then again, he would be off to another station after some time. All the time would be spent in tuning to different stations. That is how the mind works. This happens in relation to all the other senses, too – smell, taste, touch and hearing. When the senses get steady, then the *prana,* which is shaking inside becomes steady, too. You would have noticed that, if your *prana* is unsteady before doing *pranayama,* it becomes steady once you complete it. Observe the *prana* at all those moments when you are not feeling so good or are fearful. The matter may not be serious but the *prana* will be shaking. *Samadhi* is steadiness in the *prana.* However, you should not worry if the *prana* is shaking. You should not shake with the *prana.* You should just know, observe and be with it for a few moments, and the *prana* becomes steady. This is centeredness, and it brings you to a space where you are completely hollow and empty.

In this sutra Patanjali said that one becomes like a crystal. A crystal exists, but it lets the light pass through it totally. Though you exist with a body, in the state of *samadhi* you are not there at all. In other words, you can live as though you do not exist. This is *samadhi*. When you are with the Self, you are just with the Self - steady, blissful and joyful. And when you are with the senses, you are totally with the senses. When you are with the object of the senses, you become the object of the senses. This is what happens in a crystal. If you keep a coloured light behind a crystal, then the crystal, without any obstruction, assumes the colour of the light. In the same way, if you look at a mountain and become one with the mountain, it is *samadhi*.

Patanjali said that there were two types of *Samadhi*. One is the *samadhi* which you experience during activity. That is *sabeeja samadhi*. You have often done this as a child. Have you noticed a child? Its eyes are not flitting here and there. They are very steady. A child stares at things and there is a depth in its eyes. This indicates steadiness and stability of the soul. The eyes are the windows for you to see the world and the world to see your soul; to see its steadiness. If someone is very ambitious and greedy, their eyes will indicate it. The eyes of a person, who is kind and compassionate, reflect that. Eyes represent the face, the senses, the behaviour and everything else. Your appearance, your walk, your behaviour, your words and your entire life reflects what you are deep inside. This is the job of the senses.

It gives you the knowledge of the world. When you polish this and make yourself hollow and empty, you become like a crystal. The soul in you reflects the divinity, the Lord. The senses in you reflect that soul, that Lordship in you. Then, when you look at a flower, you are not just looking at it. You are touching it, feeling the flower and listening to it. All your senses become totally active. The being in you, your senses and the object of your senses, reflect one divinity like the crystal. This reflects the *purusha* in you. This is *sabeeja samadhi*. You look at a mountain and it reminds you of the Self, the consciousness. You look at a flower and the flower reminds you of consciousness. You look at the sun, moon, water, etc and that gives you the idea of the formless energy, the Self, by which all of it had come up. And at that very moment you are in *samadhi*. You may be looking at a sunset and then you are in *samadhi* because the mind and the senses are steady. Steadiness is dignity. Steadiness is strength. It is dispassion.

You can experiment. For a few moments, keep your body and your eyes steady and you will see, almost immediately, the mind will also become steady. If you stand still, the mind will become still and the breath will become steady. This is when the time stops, death stops and immortality begins. You wake up before time swallows you and before this earth gulps you. Then, you swallow time. This is *samadhi*. *Samadhi* is that state where you feel you can stay like that for a million years. It is a state where the mind freezes. It is just like things remaining fresh, if they are put in a fridge. *Samadhi* is the refrigerator of your life. It is the secret of youthfulness, the secret of bubbling enthusiasm and the secret of renewal of life. It is steadiness. But we have the wrong understanding of *samadhi*. We think it means going underground and not breathing. People in *samadh*i fast and become very skinny. They apply ash all over their body. They have wrong ideas about it.

When you are in *Samadhi*, every experience of your senses becomes very bright, colourful and complete. When you are happy, you feel expanded. You feel as if you are bloated. Something in you is expanding. You are not aware of your body, but you feel an expansion taking place. And what happens when you feel sad? You feel uptight and sorrowful. There seems to be a contraction, tightness or reduction in you. And when you feel expanded and your awareness is expanding, you tend to fall asleep. And when you want to have a keenness of awareness, you seem to be more uptight and not relaxed. It takes alertness to thread a needle. A drowsy or drunk person cannot do it. If they have to string very small pearls, they cannot do it. It needs keenness of awareness to do something very minute. There are many people who are very skillful. They can carve things on one grain of rice. They have a lot of sharpness of awareness. At the same time, when the awareness is expanded, there is no keenness of awareness. When there is keenness of awareness, there is no relaxation; there is no expansion of awareness. The combination of both of these is *sabeeja samadhi* - when you are totally relaxed, happy and expanded and when, at the same time, you have that sharpness of awareness and sharpness of intelligence. Your senses become so clear that it can perceive better, see better, think better, hear better. Ninety-five percent of the population in the world cannot hear properly. If you tell people something and ask them to repeat it, you can bet that they will not be able to do it. Or, if you talk to them for fifteen minutes and ask them to repeat what you said, they will hardly be able to repeat what you said for one minute at the most. What you had said in the rest of the time has just passed them by. They have not heard it.

This happens with sight, too. People are not able to see things as they are. We are insensitive to people's feelings because we do not see or hear properly.

Samadhi is being sensitive to other's feelings too. When you become sensitive, the world and the nature becomes sensitive to you. Nature listens to you. How can this happen? What is the condition?

Patanjali says, "*Ksheena vritti.*" When all these five activities that we have dealt with before, when these *vrittis*, the activities are subdued.

क्षीणवृत्तेरभिजातस्येवमणेर्ग्रहीतृग्रहणग्राह्येषु तत्स्थतदञ्जनता समापत्तिः

Ksheena vrittih abhijaatasya evamaneh graheetu grahana graahyeshu tatstha tadanjanataa samaapattih.

When the consciousness which grabs or holds, the object which it holds and the senses through which it holds are in harmony, there is *samadhi*. The one who is seeing, the mind, the Self, which is seeing, is in harmony. The senses are in harmony.

The eyes are the instruments through which you hold the scene. The ears are the instrument through which you hear the sound. Your ears, the sound that is heard and its source are connected. They all become keen, crystal clear. When can this happen? This can happen when your mind is not going on its own trip of regret, anger, anticipation, sleep, the five *vrittis* – proof, wrong knowledge, fantasy, sleep and memory. When you look at a mountain, you just don't look at it as it is. Something is added to it. You are not seeing things as they are, but you are seeing them through your memory, seeing through comparison. That is no *samadhi*.

There is an old story in India. A king heard about a beautiful sunflower garden that a person had made in a desert in Rajasthan. Everybody said that it was very beautiful and that he should see it. So, he decided to go there. There he saw just one flower. The person had removed all the others. The king was surprised. Then, the person offered that one flower for the king to see. He said that if there were many flowers, the king would begin to compare. His calculating mind would start wondering which was the biggest, which had blossomed and which had not, etc. So, he had removed all the other flowers to make it easy for the king. Now, he has no choice. He could look at only one flower.

Graheeta grahana graahyeshu. *Graheeta* – that which holds -the mind, the soul; that which is held - the sight, sound, taste, memory, and through which it holds - the senses and the object; - all the three are in harmony.

That is *sampattihi.* *Tatastha tadanjanataa.* Though you are engaged in the activities of the senses, there is no feverishness. There is a steadiness. You may be eating food. You taste every bit of it and it is just moving smoothly down your throat. When you are not steady, you will just stuff the food inside you. It will be like a stampede. The more anxious, nervous or shaky that you are, the faster will you stuff food into yourself. This is not *samadhi.* You should eat food thoroughly. Sixty percent of the food gets digested in the saliva in the mouth.

Tatra shabda artha jnaana vikalpaha sankeerna savitarka samapattihi.

You should have steadiness despite being in any sensory activity.

And, then Patanjali went on to explain about the very subtle modification of the senses. You may be experiencing something. Even here, the mind comes up with some knowledge about it – that it is an apple that you are eating. Or, that it is a rose that you are seeing and so on. All this is a very subtle discussion, or awareness of the knowledge of the past and the future. Patanjali called it *savitarka*. In this state, there is little debate and few thoughts come and go. But these thoughts have not disturbed the harmony. There are certain thoughts that do not disturb the harmony and certain ones that throw you off balance. There are certain thoughts that help you to arrive at that steady and calm state of awareness. Patanjali said that that was *savitarka samadhi* - when there are some thoughts or discussions.

स्मृतिपरिशुद्धौ स्वरुपशून्येवार्थमात्रनिर्भासा निर्वितर्का

Smriti parishuddhau swaroopa shoonyaiva artha maatra nirbhaasa nirvitarkaa.

And there is another type of *samadhi*, when you are not aware of anything. You just know that you are. That is it. This meditation is done with the eyes closed. When your eyes are closed, you just know that you are. But you do not know where you are, what you are or who you are - as though you are not there at all. There is just an *aabhas*, a feeling that you are nothing more than the feeling that "I am."

Patanjali called this *nirvichara samadhi, nirvitarka samadhi.*

The other types of *Samadhi* are finer and finer aspects of this.

निर्विचारवैशारद्येऽध्यात्मप्रसादः

Nirvichaara vaishaaradye adhyaatma prasaadah.

More and more experience of the thoughtless state of mind brings *adhyaatma prasaadaha* – grace of the divine in life. Grace of the soul gets manifested in you. *Adhyaatma prasaadaha.* There is spiritual awakening and blossoming. You become more and more hollow and empty.

Nirvichaara vaishaaraadye – mastery over hollow and emptiness. *Nirvichaara*, means hollow and empty. *Adhyaatma prasaadaha* – the grace of the being, the innermost comes forth and blossoms.

ऋतम्भरा तत्र प्रज्ञा

Ritambharaa tatra pragyaa.

This awareness comes about with a special knowledge. *Ritambharaa* – intuitive knowledge - the knowledge which is flawless, steady, benevolent and beyond time. *Ritambharaa* - full of truth. *Ritambharaa tatra prajnaa* - True state of consciousness.

And it is different from

श्रुतानुमानप्रज्ञाभ्यामन्यविषया विशेषार्थत्वात्

Shruta anumana pragyaabhyaam anya vishayaa vishesha

arthatvaat.

The knowledge which comes from the depth of the being is different from one which you acquire or which you have heard of or which you can guess through your intellect. *Shrutanumana pragnaabhyaam anya vishayaa vishesha arthavaat.* It is different, and very special.

तज्जः संस्कारोऽन्यसंस्कारप्रतिबन्धी

Tajjah samsakaaroh anya sanskaara pratibhandhi.

The impression of that state of consciousness can wipe out all other impressions in the mind which are useless and not necessary for life. This happens to some extent with all - maybe five, ten, fifteen, twenty, fifty or eighty percent. Something of the past is erased in your first meditation. You begin to feel that you are a new person the deeper you go and more hollow and empty that you become. You feel you are a different person. Many have had this experience. What has happened is that other *samskaras* and impressions have been erased from your mind. It has made you new. It renews you again, and again, and again, and again. Often, when you have thought of events in the past, you would have felt that you are not the same person that you were then. You even feel that it was not you at all; as though you are not at all connected to those events. This is because this *samskara* of your consciousness has been erasing those things of your past continuously and has been making you a new person every day.

This is pure knowledge. If someone holds you to something you did in the past, you should laugh at them. This is because you are not the same person now. You should see it as if somebody else had done it.

Once Buddha was in an assembly and a gentleman came to him. He was furious. He thought that Buddha was doing something wrong. He was attracting people and everybody had begun meditating. The people had become very calm and quiet. The gentleman was a restless businessman. He had found that his children were going and sitting with Buddha and meditating for two hours every day. And he thought that if his children would be engaged in business, they could make more money and be better off. What would they get by sitting for two hours with somebody with their eyes closed? So he was angry and wanted to teach a Buddha a lesson.

He walked up to Buddha but as soon as he came near him all his thoughts disappeared. But he was still shaking with anger and could not speak. No words would come out of his mouth. So he spat on Buddha's face. And Buddha just smiled. However, all the other disciples there became furious but could not react because Buddha was there. So, everybody restrained themselves.

The man could not stay any longer because he thought that if he stayed any longer, he would burst out. He went away. He could not sleep the whole night. For the first time in his life, he had met somebody who would just smile when he spat on his face. He began shivering. His world had turned topsy-turvy.

The next day he went to Buddha fell at his feet. He asked for forgiveness and said that he was not aware of what he had done. However, Buddha said that he could not forgive him. The disciples were shocked to hear this. Buddha was so compassionate and forgave everybody. How could he not forgive that person! But Buddha explained that the person had done nothing for which forgiveness was required. However, the person pointed out that he was the same person who had spat on Him the previous day. Then, Buddha said that, that person was not there anymore and, if he ever met him, he would forgive. Further, Buddha pointed out that the person had done no wrong to the man standing before him.

That is compassion.

Compassion is not making a person a culprit and then forgiving him. Your forgiveness should be such that the person, who is being forgiven, does not even know that you are forgiving them. They should not even feel guilty of a mistake. That is the right type of forgiveness. If you make someone feel guilty about their mistake, then you have not forgiven them. That guilt itself is the punishment. It is good enough to eat the wrongdoer. Knowledge takes you away from guilt and puts you on a pedestal where you do not see the world at all. You do not see the world of the small mind and its chitchat. It appears insignificant.

तस्यापि निरोधे सर्वनिरोधान्निर्बीजः समाधिः साधनपादः

Tasyapi nirodhe sarva nirodhaannirbeejah samadhih saadhnpaadah.

This is another kind of *samadhi* where even the feeling of some impressions is not there. There is no end to this. There are many different states of awareness and types of *samadhi* being described. The path is long. Every step is complete in itself. It is not that you are aiming at a goal after sometime. The goal is in every moment. Yet the path is long. The path is very long, yet the goal is there at every moment. The goal is where you are. You are not in a hurry and want *samadhi* immediately. There should be enthusiasm and along with it there should be patience. Those who are very enthusiastic have no patience. People who have patience are very lethargic. There is either one extreme or the other. You can sleep but you cannot have a quick sleep. Hurried sleep is not possible. You cannot feel that, since you are in a hurry, you should sleep quickly and then rise and go. In the same way, you cannot remember something in a hurry. This hurry delays it all the more. It is the same with the meditation. If you do not have the time, you cannot have a quick meditation. So this path is a middle path, a golden path, wherein you are enthusiastic and are in a hurry but, at the same time, you are patient. You are patient and, at the same time, you are not lethargic. You are not postponing things. Often, if people have to do something good, something for their personal development, they will feel that, if God is willing, they will do it and it will happen. They leave it to God when it comes to their practices and development. But if they have to do something in the world, they do not leave it to God. They will not, if they have to build a house or have a relationship. They will put in their hundred percent for that. So, patience and dynamism is the golden rule.

Chapter 7

KRIYA YOGA

When someone is anxious, they are very aware of the passage of time; of every moment. However, then the total focus is on an event or a happening rather than just on time. Someone may be waiting for a train, a bus or a boat and they will go on thinking if it is coming. The focus is on the concerned object rather than just on the time.

But, if there is a little shift done by you, then when you wait for somebody or something, you will just wait for the moment – for "Now". This is uniting with the time. This is Yoga. When you do this, you mind is in the moment and waiting for nothing. However, you are still waiting. This adds a different quality to the consciousness. It sharpens the intellect and softens the heart. This is called the Yoga of action.

This is the next sutra in Patanjali's second chapter, *Sadhana Pada*.

Sadhana Pada means, the path of practice.

तप: स्वाध्यायेश्वरप्रणिधानानि क्रियायोग:

Tapah swaadhyaaya ishwara pranidhaanani kriya yogah.

Tapaha swaadhyaaya ishwara pranidhaana is *Kriya Yoga.*

Kriya Yoga is the Yoga of action. Action is part of this creation. There is activity in everything in creation - from an atom to the sun, moon and the stars. The entire creation is activity. There is nothing that is stable or immobile in this creation.

The *Brahman,* the infinity is filled with infinite activity. There is absolutely no silence at all. There is activity even in sleep. You may think that, when you are asleep, there is no activity. However, there is tremendous activity then. Your body grows more during sleep than during wakefulness. That is why a growing child sleeps longer. A youth sleeps more than an aged person because there is a lot of metabolic activity in a youth. The body is getting built up in a child. Every cell is multiplying and in sleep the cells multiply more. If you deprive somebody of sleep, their growth gets stunted.

Even in silence, there is activity. At the same time, in every activity there is a corner that is very silent.

Krishna asked Arjuna if he knew who was really intelligent. When he said that he did not, Krishna said that a person who saw silence in activity and activity in silence was intelligent. How do you see silence in activity and activity in silence? It needs sharpness of awareness, alertness and keenness. And this can be there when there is skill in your activity. Yoga is the skill in activity.

Kriya Yoga, the Yoga of action has three parts. The first is *tapaha. Tapas* is endurance and acceptance. You may be taking a long flight. You may be sitting in your seat and your legs would be getting numb. You may be feeling tired and heavy but you keep sitting. You cannot say that you will not sit anymore and that you will get out of the plane. If the plane is delayed or held up in the air, you just have to continue to be on it. There is no choice for you. Now, if you had a choice, you would not sit in one place for eight hours the way you sit on a long flight. But in a plane you accept the inevitable and sit – willingly and without grumbling. This is *tapaha. Tapaha* is experiencing the opposite values, willingly and without grumbling. You may be driving to some place at night. You are feeling sleepy as it is the time to sleep. But, you do not park somewhere and sleep. Of course, you may do this if the sleep is too heavy and there is a chance of you falling asleep while driving. Normally, you will carry on.

In the same way, one day you may decide to fast in order to cleanse you body. You may feel hungry but you will not have anything other than fruit juice and water on that day. This is *tapaha.*

You may know that the benefits of certain actions, and will want to do them - like doing exercises. People go to gymnasiums for this. The exercises do not give them any pleasure. They do not enjoy lifting weights but they do it because they know that it is good for their system. This endurance is called *tapaha.*

Tapas.

Swadhyaaya is being alert in self-study - observing one's breath and emotions. It is wondering where the thoughts and emotions come from and what happens inside you – observing and studying yourself.

Eshwara pranidhaana is devotion to and love for the Divine.

These three things together make up *Kriya Yoga*. What do they do to you?

Klesha tanu karanaarthascha – they reduce the suffering and misery in life. *Samadhi bhaavana arthaha* – this gives rise to *samadhi* – equanimity.

There are certain people who walk without wearing shoes in very hot weather. It may seem to be self-torture. But, they are used to it and, moreover, their bodies are much stronger. They can bear that heat. But it will be very unbearable for someone else.

So, *tapas* makes you strong in some areas. If a Californian goes to Switzerland, he may need to wear two sweaters and a coat. But if somebody from the North-West province, Quebec goes there, the cold will seem insignificant. He may not even need a sweater because his body is used to harsher conditions. *Tapas* is willingly doing something that is not very easy. This strengthens you. But, people can stretch this beyond proportions. They can become masochists and torture themselves. And here, too, there are three types of *tapas* – *tapas* for the body, *tapas* for the words, for speech and *tapas* in the mind.

Three Types of Tapas

Fire sustains life. There are five types of fire. One is *bhootaagni*. *Bhootaagni* is the fire with which you heat your homes and keep yourself warm. This physical fire sustains life. It may not be so obvious in tropical countries. They don't give much importance to fire. But, it is very important in cold countries. Without physical fire, life gets extinguished. And this physical fire is present in the body to some extent.

And then, there is the second type of fire which is called *kaamaagni*. This is the fire of desire, lust or passion. This fire will engulf you. Life continues on this planet because of this fire. The fire of passion is present in all the species of creation. Now, you do not even allow this fire of passion to come up in you. The moment there is a desire, you fulfil it. Then that desire does not stay in you, it doesn't burn you up. People who are very promiscuous have no *kaamaagni*. This is because they do not even allow the fire to come up and burn and bake them a little bit. The moment there is a desire for sex, they fulfill it. Then the *kaamaagni* does not get awakened in them. Sex is one of the oldest *samskaras* after eating. In all your lifetimes, you have certainly done two things – eating and sex. These two acts have been done as a cow, a monkey, a donkey, a horse or an ox. When this passion arises, observe it. It is in every cell of your body. It engulfs you totally. It burns and moves on. There is one hundred percent totality of alertness and awareness. But if you do not allow it to come up then there is a little desire. And, immediately it is cooled down. Then, your power or *shakti*, the potentiality in you goes down and becomes dormant. And you become more inert and less sensitive. There is no vigour, valour, joy, or enthusiasm in anything that you do. This is the reason that people who are very promiscuous do not have much enthusiasm. They do not have the force, will or strength to do anything. *Kaamaagni*.

The third type of fire is called *jataraagni* - the fire of hunger and digestion. This is one of the important principles in Ayurveda – *Jataraagni*. If the fire of digestion is less or more, it affects your health and your balance. When there is fever, we just treat the symptoms. We do not understand the principles involved. When a foreign body enters your body, it turns up the heat and there is fever. During a fever, your body is operating its defence mechanism. It is burning up all the foreign bacteria and viruses that have entered it. As soon as they are destroyed, the fever comes down. It purifies the system by getting rid of the foreign matter. *Jataraagni* – fire of digestion.

You don't even allow hunger to come up in you. You keep stuffing things into yourself even before you are hungry. This makes you more toxic and your body is affected. Many people get disease or die because of overeating and not of hunger. Nowadays, very few people die of hunger. However, more and more people die of overeating, because they have not let the fire of hunger come up. We have never kindled that fire. This is the principle of fasting. When you fast, every cell of your body becomes alive. It is a very good therapy. It can cleanse your system. The *jataraagni* can cleanse you of all toxins. When your head is clogged with worry, tension and unpleasant thoughts or nightmares, fasting is a very great help.

Much research has been done on fasting. You should fast and allow the *jataraagni* to come up in you. It can purify your blood and remove toxins from your body. It can help you feel better. Fasting and prayers are linked in Christianity, Jainism, Islam, and in almost all the religions of the world. This is because fasting touches the deepest *samskara*, or impression present in you from ages - to eat, eat, and just eat. There are some people who just go on fasting without being aware of the connected factors; too much fire also can burn you down. Fasting should be done with an understanding. There are people who go to extremes. Either they overeat or fast too much. Neither is good. Fasting, with moderation and guidance can cleanse your system and bring balance.

Next is the fire of knowledge or love - *Premaagni* or *jnaanaagni*.

When life will move through all these fires, it will emerge as gold. Unfortunately, you have not understood this principle. You do not even allow the fire to come up in you. When you have fever, you take paracetamol and suppress it. You just get rid of the symptoms of the problem. You do not attend to the root cause. It is not that you should not take medicines. You should take it the natural way. You should attend to the root cause of the problem and eliminate the bacteria, rather than just eliminate the symptoms or the fire in the system.

Naturopathy and *Ayurveda* deal with this principle – to keep alive the *bhootaagni*. Your body has its own air-conditioning system. But, if you turn on the external air-conditioner all the time, then you are destroying the self-modulating system of the body. The air-conditioner is kept switched on all the time in hot and tropical countries. There is no *prana*, or freshness in such an environment. When it is hot, you sweat and this cools you, just as you feel cool when there is a breeze. The body has its own air-conditioning system. But, you need to get used to this from early in life. If you have been used to air-conditioners from then, you may find it difficult to change. But nevertheless you can try. I have nothing against air-conditioners but making sure that the fresh *prana* comes and your body temperature agrees with the environment will make a difference. Then, you gain the ability to be in a cold place without having to wear too many warm clothes. Or to be in a hot place and not feel suffocated.

Then, there is *Badabaagni* – the fire of criticism. When people criticize you, there is a fire which flares up in your system. When you speak before a big crowd, you are uncomfortable and nervous because you fear their opinions and criticism. *Badabaagni* is the fire of social criticism. It is said that man is a social animal and lives in a society. He has to follow certain rules and cannot live as he pleases. He cannot feel that, since he is free, he can do whatever that he wishes. When you drive, you have to follow the rules. You have to drive on the correct side. When you walk, you have to do so in the proper place. You have to stop where you should stop. You have to follow certain rules and regulations; certain code of conduct. This will give rise to certain fears in you – the fear of criticism, the fear of getting a ticket, the fear of being punished, etc. Abiding by certain laws brings up certain concerns for keeping to those laws. If you are greatly concerned about criticism and other people's opinions about you, then you are missing the boat. Certainly, the fear of criticism keeps you within the limits of morality. But if it goes out of control or out of limit, the same fear of criticism can shut down your freedom, openness and centeredness. If the fire of criticism is too much, then you will be tensed and worried about nothing. You should pass through the fear of criticism. It does not matter what people say. Their opinions change. And you know in your consciousness that you are not doing any harm to anybody.

Then, you will move on to the fire of love – love creates such a fire in you. The fire of love can really lift you up from the fear of criticism. The fire of love is so strong that you do not mind people's opinions. It takes you totally. The fire of knowledge and the fire of love are the same. They are synonymous. Fire of love begins with a longing - an intense longing. It feels so new that it can also feel uncomfortable. This fire can be experienced only in human life, in human birth. Fire of love or fire of knowledge creates an unpleasant sense of longing in the beginning. But, then it moves on to the blossom of bliss, the blossom of fullness. These are the five fires in life – *panchaagni*.

Tapa means being fried or baked. You would have read about the *Kumbhamela* in some magazines. In this religious gathering, somebody may be standing on one leg with ashes all over his body and having a pot of fire on his head. There have been such misinterpretations of *panchaagni*.

Patanjali had said that one who will go through the five fires will be purified; would have crossed to the other side. But, the scriptures have been wrongly understood. People thought that one who passed through five actual fires would be purified. So, they lit fires all around. They started fire-walking and began to torture their bodies. This is called *rakshasitapas*.

There are three types of *tapas - sattvic, rajasic,* and *tamasic.*

Sattvic tapas is one in which you are not even aware that you are doing it. You are just part of the phenomenon. The world today is a phenomenon and you are just a part of that phenomenon. Where do you exist? There may be so many waves or ripples in a lake but it is ridiculous if each one of them thinks that it is existing as a wave. When a wind blows, so many waves arise, and they all subside a little later. Similarly, in the ocean of consciousness, many waves have arisen. And one wave calls itself Jyothi, another is Michel, and there would be others - David, Dev and Lillian. Those limited waves have been given different names. And all these waves will subside in a few years, and new waves will arise. One goes through this fire of life with this awareness. This is *sattvic tapas.*

Rajasic- there are those who do practices with a desire to achieving something. They have this motive even when they are doing some service or *seva.* And, this has a mixed effect. This is *rajasic tapas* - the *tapas* a person does to show off. One may fast, meditate or do great service but broadcast it, as well. So the *tapas* is done with pomp and show; with much 'I'-ness.

Tamasic is the demonic *tapas,* where people torture themselves, because they cannot torture others. If you torture yourself, nobody will question you. They put nails all over the body and walk on fire.

There are three other sections of *tapas* - the bodily *tapas*, the *tapas* of the speech, and *tapas* of the mind.

Bodily *tapas* is maintaining physical hygiene, avoiding lethargy, having control over the five senses, etc. You may want to watch the television, but you do not. You are not hungry and you just do not eat even if you want to. Physical *tapas* is maintaining personal hygiene and continence, remaining in the Self and having a control over the senses and the body.

And then, there is *tapas* of the speech. This is saying only such things that do not distress people - speaking the truth and speaking the pleasant truth – *anudwega karm vakyam charit satyam, priyam hitam*. Make a note of what you tell people when you are with them; what do you talk about? Do you excite them and do they leave you feeling relieved and at peace or do they leave you feeling angry, jealous, greedy, frustrated or depressed? Often, you are a better person when you are silent. You are more charming and likeable. You will be wanted more. However, you may have no control over what you say and words just come shooting out of your mouth. You may not even think about their effects; how they can be like daggers in somebody's mind. Your words can become a flower or a knife.

Vangmaya tapas – those words that do not ruffle people's calm and quiet mind. It is different if you want to intentionally disturb another person. But often, what you say creates a disturbance in others' minds and it is unintentional. This is *vangmaya tapas*. Those who speak harshly feel that they are saying the truth. They feel that there is no need to skirt the truth. However, what is said can be pleasant expressions of truth. An example is often given in Sanskrit. If you meet someone who is blind, you can call him to you by addressing him as one. Granted, it a truth that you are saying. But doing so can greatly hurt the person. Instead you can address him as *Prajnachakshu*. This implies his third eye which is his consciousness. In Sanskrit, this is often quoted as an example of speaking sweetly – calling a blind person a man of consciousness or someone who sees with his third eye of consciousness – someone with intuitive eyes. This is *vangmaya tapas*.

Vangmaya tapas is important because as you grow in this path of Yoga – your words become more, and more, and more powerful. You may call someone a fool. And, even if he is not a fool, he will become one. So your words will have the power to bless as well as curse. *Vangmaya tapas* purifies you. Otherwise those things rebound back to you. If you speak harshly, your words will affect you adversely. This does not mean that you should ever be goody-goody. That is also self-deception. You do not have to be a split person ie. be outwardly nice and cordial and be just the opposite inside. Then again, you do not need to be a harsh expresser of truth. This is *vangmaya tapas*.

And then there is *manomaya tapas* - *tapas* of the mind.

Manaha prasaadaha sowmyataam mounam aatma vinigraha.

Patanjali has said four things.

Manaha prasaadaha – the pleasantness in the mind. It is a big tapas to maintain the pleasantness of the mind. You may feel pleasant but soon you drop all that pleasantness. *Manaprasaadah* - maintaining the pleasantness and contentment in the mind.

Sowmyataam. Sowmya means calm and composed. You can feel pleasant, but excited. That is not *sowmya*. Some people feel very pleasant but they do not feel calm. The pleasantness can make them feel very crazy and excited. So, along with pleasantness it is essential to be composed - *sowmyataam.* People who are happy create trouble for others. This is because they are not aware that, in their excitement and happiness, they say and do things that may adversely affect others. But if a person is calm and composed, he is more aware. There is awareness in a composed mind. You are sensitive to others' feelings and to your surroundings. So, what is required is a pleasant and composed mind. *Manaha prasaadaha sowmyataam.*

Mounam – a silent mind; not a chattering mind. Silence is the *tapas* of the mind. *Mounam* is the silence obtained by bringing together the scattered mind and tying all the loose ends.

Aatma vinigraha – remaining in the Self; getting back to the Self. This is the *tapas* of the mind. The mind loses its way again and again. It needs to be brought back to the Self.

And see the Self in everybody. Feel this person is also you and that person, too – everybody. Normally, we think our mind is in the body. But it is not so. The body is inside the mind. Your body of *prana* is ten times bigger than your physical body. Your energy, bio-energy is ten times bigger than the physical body. And ten times bigger than the *pranic* body is your mind body, your thought body. And ten times bigger than that is your intuitive body. And ten times bigger than that is the blissful body. Our blissful body is boundless. That is why when you feel blissful and happy you do not feel any boundary. You feel expanded and do not feel any limit to yourself. And when you feel sad or unhappy, you feel crushed, because then your *prana* is getting smaller than your real body. This is the mechanism of unhappiness. It is like trying to put your body through a small hole where it cannot fit. This is the reason why you feel so unhappy. When you try to crush your *prana*, which is so big into a small space, you feel unhappy. Whenever you are unhappy in life, know that you have put your love into a small channel. Your love is so great, so big. It needs a royal door to walk through. But you have stuck that big elephant-body of your love, into a small chimney, or ventilator. It can neither go out nor come in. This is entanglement. That is why that love seems to bring problems to you. You do not understand its magnitude.

This is *tapas. Manomaya tapas. Aatma vinigraha* - coming back to the Self, holding to the centeredness in you.

Chapter 8

THE VEILS OF MISERY

We are talking about *tapas*. What does *tapas* do? Why should we undergo *tapas*?

It purifies our system and strengthens our system – purity and strength. That is the purpose of *tapas*. But *tapas* can bring a big ego in a person. Unfortunately, people think by doing *tapas*, they will become very great. If someone has to fast for long periods of time, he must have had lots of impurities. Out of proportion glorification of *tapas* leads to ego.

That is why the next thing to be done immediately after *tapas* is swaadhyaaya. *Swaadhyaaya* is self-study. Why do you fast? Is it just to show off? Is it in competition with somebody?

There is a story. There were two persons who were meditating and doing some tapas. They were neighbours. And, God came to one of them and asked him what he wanted. The man said that he wanted whatever He would give to his neighbour.

He asked God if He was visiting his neighbour, too. God replied that he certainly would, considering that both of them had started *tapas* on the same day. God pointed out that He had come there first because he had started his *tapas* an hour earlier. He again asked the man what he wanted. The man asked Him if He could avoid going to his neighbour. God refused, saying that it would be an injustice if He did so. He had to go there. God, once again, asked the man what he wanted. The man replied that he wanted twice as much of whatever God gave the other man.

Then God went to the other man and asked him what he wanted. He asked if He had not come to him after seeing his neighbour. God said that He had. The man asked God what He had given to his neighbour. Initially, God was silent. When the man insisted, He said that the neighbour had asked to be given twice as much of whatever he would want. And the man asked God to take away one of his eyes, and one of his ears. That would teach his neighbour a lesson. Continuing, he said that the neighbour was always in competition with him. And God could give him twice as much as he had been given.

This sort of *tapas,* without self-study, leads to ego. So immediately, almost in the same sutra, Patanjali has said, "*Swaadhyaaya*" – self-study.

Look into the motives behind your actions. Often, you do not go for things that you really want. You go for them because others want them. You may even go for something depending on what others would say, think or do about it. And many times you are not clear about what you want because you have never really looked into yourself. You are swayed by fleeting thoughts, fleeting emotions and fleeting desires. Your desire may not even be your own. Maybe, some outside factors – food, events, situations or company have raised a storm in you and you start believing that storm as your very Self. That is why often you are not happy even when your desires are fulfilled. You should observe the Self. You should wonder who you are and what you are. You have purified the body, but are you the body? You have made your mind light, but are you the mind? Are you your thoughts? Are you your emotions? Who are you? This self-study leads you upwards to the universe that is unknown to us. Self-study takes you a step further and eliminates misery and suffering of the mind.

Buddha has said this so beautifully. He said *kaayaanupaschana*, observe the body.

That is *tapas*.

Vedanaanupaschana - You should sensations in the body.

Chittaanupaschana - You should observe the mind –its impressions, thoughts and feelings.

Dhammaanupaschana – You should observe your very nature; observe the *dharma*. Buddha has said that there are four steps for this.

Patanjali has said the same thing. *Tapaha swaadhyaaya ishwara pranidhaana.*

Swaadhyaaya can eliminate all mental and emotional impurities, uncertainties, fears and anxieties and *ishwara pranidhana* – love of God and surrender to the Lord will complete the process. Without love, self-study becomes another dry stuff. Without surrender, self-study is not charming. Without love and devotion the spiritual path becomes very dry - like Styrofoam. It is like a cake or pudding without sugar; bread without salt.

Ishwara pranidhana. How can love for Lord blossom in us?

The first step is to see Lord as different from you - Lord and me. Two are needed for surrender - when you feel that there is Lord of all virtues and that you are nobody. In this nobody-ness, the union takes place. The realization dawns that all is the Lord and then that all is me, me, I, I; that the universe is the Lord's, your body is His, your mind with all its conflicts and you mind with all its beauty is also His. This offering itself is a technique which brings you back home.

Ishwara pranidhana brings about *samadhi*, or ecstasy in that meditation. Offering candles, incense or flowers is not great. You should offer every part of your body, offer every moment of life, offer every breath, offer every thought – good, bad, pleasant, unpleasant, anything. Offer all those *vasanas* or those things which you consider are your negative points. Offer all your negativity and offer all your positivity. By offering all the negativity, you become free. Offering all the positive virtues you think you posses, you become free. You will not become arrogant. Your virtues make you arrogant. They make you behave as if you are special. And your drawbacks pull you down and make you feel bad about yourself. And if you start feeling bad about yourself and unconnected to the Divine, there is nothing that can make you feel connected. It is up to you to feel close to the Divine. It is up to you to feel close to anybody for that matter. Even if they do not feel close to you, you should start feeling close. It does not matter if they do not feel that you are close to them.

And how do you know this? You cannot know just by their behaviour. It is not the right way to judge. This is because nothing else can convince you that you are close and dear to the Divine other than your own mind and your own self. You should stop comparing. This applies to the Master, too. You may feel that somebody is close to the Master because he smiles and talks more often to them. That, he does not smile at or talk to you. This is your illusion. It does not matter if the Master does not talk to you. You should start feeling you are the only one and that you are the closest to him. Then you will see that what you want will start happening; that it will start blossoming. Whatever seed you sow, that will grow. If you sow the seed that you are hopeless and no good, then that no-good seed will grow. Often, weeds and other useless things grow without any cultivation. You do not need to cultivate weeds. That is why they are called weeds. They just grow and thrive on their own. But a useful plant needs some attention. In your field many weeds are coming up every day - useless, unwanted and unnecessary doubts and thoughts. You don't need to sow them. They just come up by themselves. By *swaadhyaaya*, you can weed them out and maintain only that, which is essential in life.

तपः स्वाध्याया ईश्वरा प्राणिधानु क्रियायोगः

Tapaha swaadhyaaya ishwara pranidhaana kriya yogaha.

This is the Yoga of action. But even when you are doing something, you should think that you are not doing it. You should be a silent witness. There is a depth in you, a silent corner that does not change. All the activity is taking place in this silent space. Every atom is revolving around the nucleus and all the planets are moving around. Yet, there is silence.

The purpose of this is *klesha tanukarana* – to reduce the suffering or misery in life. *Samadhi bhaavanaarthaha* – and to bring about *samadhi*, harmony and equanimity in life.

What are the root causes of misery in life?

Avidya, asmita, raga, dwesha, abhinivesha, panchakleshaaha.

Avidya is ignorance. It is the root cause of all suffering.

Ignorance is to consider permanent that which is not so; to think or to understand that which is changing to be unchanging; that which is not joy to be joy, and which is not Self to be the Self. It is thinking you are the body when you are not; thinking that you are your thoughts and emotions when you are not. It is considering your body to be unchanging, when it is, actually, changing continuously. Doctors say that the blood is changed every twenty-four hours and in five days your stomach lining changes. And the skin changes in a month. Every cell in the body changes in a year. In a year all the old cells are dead and gone and you have new ones. Your body is new. Your mind is new. However, you have never considered your body like a river which is undergoing change all the time.

As you awaken to this truth, you will not identify with your old fears and thoughts; with the old you. Your ignorance makes you hold on to them; hold on to your past. You hold on to your idea of who you are. People think it is a very complimentary to know who you are; to have an idea about yourself. But, if you have an idea of who you are, then you get stuck. The right attitude is to feel that you do not know who you are. This is because you are changing every moment. And you have understood this process when you do not know your own identity. A fixed idea about who you are destroys you totally. It stops your growth and limits your potential.

Ignorance is considering that which is changing to be non-changing. We try to control others' mind. This is not possible. Someone may have loved you yesterday. But, they need not love you today or tomorrow. They would not know this themselves. You expect an enlightened behaviour from everybody around you and when you do not get it, you become unhappy. You may not be behaving in an enlightened way, but you expect everyone around you to be enlightened and have unconditional love for you. A person who loves you unconditionally is rare - one in a million. But you expect it from everybody around you. This expectation makes you unhappy. This is what everybody is doing, consciously or unconsciously. Sometimes, they may not even know what they are expecting. But their expectation is something very big. They are seeking God in everybody. They are seeking God without understanding that God could behave in any manner that He wants. They are looking for a saintly God in everybody around them. Your concept of how things should be makes you miserable.

Asmita is oneness of our intellect and our self. Have you noticed that some people, stubbornly, stick to their opinion despite the facts being contrary to it? They will argue meaninglessly. This happens because they are so stuck in themselves, in their intellect and thoughts, which they consider as their own. *Asmita* is the inability to see the Self and the *buddhi* or the intellect and the power of the organs of perception as separate entities.

Raga is craving. Craving arises because of a pleasant

experience and it makes you miserable. Patanjali had said that there were only five sources of misery.

अविद्यास्मितारागद्वेषाभिनिवेशाः क्लेशाः

Avidyasmitaaraagdweshaabhiniveshah kleshah

Avidya asmita raga dwesha. Dwesha is hatred. Hatred or aversion brings an unpleasant experience. Aversion brings the same misery as craving. Both craving and aversion are sources of misery.

Abhinivesha is fear – fear of the unknown. Though intellectually you may know everything, you will have a bit of *abhinivesha*. This fear exists even in scholars.

Nature has imposed these fears in everybody. If they become thin, you will be evolved and if they remain thick, you will stay unevolved.

These fears and miseries have four stages.

The first stage is when they are dormant in you.

The next sutra is *prasupta avastha*.

These miseries can be *prasupta* - asleep or dormant. *Tanu* means very feeble, almost non-existent.

Prachchinna means that when one of the miseries becomes dominant, the others subside. When there is a craving, aversion subsides. So does fear and the other miseries. And when there is *avidya* or ignorance, you are not even aware of the two things in you – you and your mind, you and your perception, your intellect. You are not aware that your mind is telling you something. You don't feel there is any difference between you and your mind. You are so totally caught up in a situation. When you are conscious and aware, then you know what your mind is telling you. You will see that difference in you. If you are conscious and aware and you do something wrong, you will wonder what has happened to you; whether you are going crazy? When a person has really become crazy, he will not even be aware that he has become so. This is because he and his mind has become one. It is unable to see the distinction. Sometimes you get angry but you are not expressing the anger. You know that you are angry and you wonder why you are so. Or you may become lustful and be aware of it. But, a person who loses his temper is not aware that he is angry. He becomes the anger.

So, *sadhana* makes these five *kleshas,* or sources of misery, as thin as possible with the passage of time. You had been getting angry before you were on the spiritual path and after, too. But there is a big difference in the quality of anger. There is a shift. After being on the spiritual path, the anger has become *tanu* – thinned down. The curtain has become more and more transparent.

Prachchinna means one is dominant and the others have all

gone underground. And *udaara*, means very generous, fully active. This you can find in the societies all over the world. All the miseries are present in their generous form in people who are not doing any practice or meditation. It is so nice of Patanjali to call them generous. There is no shortage of frustrated and miserable people all through the ages. *Udaara* is the form when they are fully active.

A little fear should be kept in the body, so that the body can be maintained. It should be lesser than salt, less than a pinch. That is why it is called *vidushoopi*. It is found even in persons who have much knowledge about scriptures.

Actually, it is not fear. It is alertness. There is a difference. Alertness implies being careful. There is a similarity between alertness and fear. That is why Patanjali has used the word *abhinivesha*, and not *bhaya* which means fear. There is no equivalent word for *Abhinivesha* in English. *Abhinivesha* in its crude form is fear and in its subtle form is care.

You may be walking on the edge of a lake. You are walking carefully so that you do not fall into the water. If this care is not there for the body, then the body could just vanish, disappear. You may feel that when you are not the body, you do need not attend to it at all. To maintain the body, a certain amount of care is essential. And when this care increases little more than what is really needed then there is insecurity. If there is a further increase, then there is fear. If it increases beyond fear it becomes paranoia. It is just like increasing the amount of salt in food. After a certain amount, it becomes impossible to eat that food.

But here, one cannot justify, saying that a bit could be there. That a little ignorance can be acceptable. *Tanu karana* – thin them down and reduce them to their minimum.

Avidya, asmita, raga, dwesha, abhinivesha, the five *kleshas,* five sources of misery.

ते प्रतिप्रसवहेयाः सूक्ष्माः

Te pratiprasavaheyaah sookshmaah.

When you make the sources of misery and the fears more and more subtle, they let you return to your Self. They let you bring the mind back to the Source. When these miseries are very thick, they bother you. They captivate your mind. When they become thinner and thinner, they begin to let your mind become free and get back to its Self, the Source. When you are craving for somebody and it is not subtle, you are unable to relax or even be still. However, once that craving is gone, then you are able to relax and meditate. The feverishness gets reduced and the mind can get back to the Source.

Now, what is the way to get rid of these miseries in life?

The next *sutra* is *Dhyaana heyas tadvrittayaha.*

These five *vrittis* can be eliminated through meditation. Misery can be overcome through meditation. Patanjali emphasized that it could be done only through meditation. If you do not do it, then what will happen?

क्लेशमूलः कर्माशयो दृष्टादृष्टजन्मवेदनीयः

Klesha moolah karmaashayo drishta adrishta janma vedaneeyah.

If you don't cleanse your consciousness of these five miseries or impurities, then you will have to suffer in this life and the next, too.

Patanjali said *drishtaadrishta janma vedaneeyaha* - you will have to suffer in this life and in the next life too, because the miseries form *karmaashaya* - a bank of *karma*. They get into the reserve bank in you. They form a *karma* tank. This *karma* can be washed off and eliminated right away through meditation. You should get rid of the *karma* and lessen the sheaths of ignorance over you before your body drops. Otherwise, there is no escape for you from these miseries.

Drishtaadrishta janma vedaniyaha.

Some karma will give you fruit in this life and some in the next. Some people may ask, if one day you put your finger in the fire, whether it will burn that day, the next day, the next year or in the next lifetime. They will point out that there is nothing like *karma.* They will agree that every action has its repercussions, which are felt in the current lifetime, itself. That it does not come with you to the next life. Some people have this argument. But it is not correct. Different seeds have different periods for sprouting. Alfalfa sprouts in three days, peanuts in four days to five days and coconut may take several months. If you plant lettuce, you can use it for salads in two to three months. If you plant mango it will give you fruit in ten years; avocado in four, five years, seven years. If you plant a jackfruit, only the next generation will enjoy the fruit. Different fruits and vegetables have got different time periods to give fruit.

Likewise, different *karmas* will give fruits at different times. Many people ask why bad things happen to good people. Bad things never happen to good people. They may be good at present. But they have done something bad in the past, so they are getting the result for it. It is as if they had planted *neem* seeds long ago. So now, they reap the bitter fruit of *neem* tree. Currently, they may be sowing mango. They will have sweet mangoes in the future. As you sow, so shall you reap. *Drishtaadrishta janma vedaniyaaha.*

सतिमुले तद्विपाको जात्यार्युभोगः

Sati mole tadwipaako jaatyaayurbhoogaaha.

Patanjali explains a little more about the genesis, and how we gain our birth. As long as this root is there, the fruit of its tree will grow again and again.

Jaatyaayurbhoogaaha. Jaati means the body in which there is birth. The birth may be as a chicken, or a monkey, or a human – or a male or a female. Your birth and the length of your life is determined. What you will get in your life, your enjoyments, or sufferings are also determined. Why is someone born in Ethiopia and someone else in Switzerland? Why is one person born in one place and another is born somewhere else? Why is one person miserable? Why is another, who has done nothing wrong, suffering? No logic can give you any understanding or explanation.

Patanjali had an insight into this phenomenon. He said the current birth of a person is due to past *karmas – jaatyaayur bhoga.* It comes to you in different forms. If a person dies with memories of chicken and if the strongest impression at the moment of death was a chicken, he will be reborn as one. The strongest impression in the mind at the time of death persists. At night, just before going to bed, think of something. Think very strongly about it. And as soon as you wake up in the morning, that will be your first thought. And at night, it will be dreamt of, too. And if you practice it for some time you will assume those qualities in you. You may think that, as soon as you wake up, you should shake your head like your dog. In six months, you will begin to do it and it will be out of control because it influences you so deeply; because that *karma*, that impression has become so strong. If you keep watching a dog and that image keeps coming in your mind all the time. Your mind and consciousness gets sucked into that type of body when you die. So it is said that the last days of life are much more important than the whole life.

There are so many stories in India to emphasize this. Usually an old man is very attached to his children. They name their children after the various gods.

There is a story about a King Ajamila. Ajamila was a king who was an atheist till his death. At the last moment when he was dying, he thought of his son and called out for him. His son's name was Narayana. It seems God thought he was being called, so Narayana came and liberated him. It is an exaggerated way to say that the last impression carries much weight.

There is a similar story about a saint who was very enlightened. One day, he was meditating on the bank of a river which was in flood. He saw a baby deer being carried away in the flood. So he jumped in and saved it, like any human would do. He bandaged its wounds and cared for it. He got very attached to it. And it is said that after he died he became a deer in his next birth. It is said that it is almost impossible for a liberated man to go back into an animal body. This example is quoted just to indicate that the last impression is very important. This happens when you go to sleep. If children see horror movies before going to bed at night, they have nightmares. How do you get rid of this?

ते ह्लृदपरितापफलाः पुण्यापुण्यहेतुत्वात्

Te haldaparitaapa phalaah punya apunya hetutwaat.

When these impressions are good, they bring you much joy and happiness. However, if they not good, they bring suffering. It depends on your merit and demerit. If you have done good to people, then that good *karma* accumulates and brings you joy. If somebody is happy, it is because he has done something good in the past. If somebody is miserable, he has done something bad in the past. So, here Patanjali connects every happiness and misery to some action of the past - all that is in your *karma* tank.

And, meditation is the way we wash out the misery. You become so light, hollow and empty. You sing and dance to make thin the veil which is on the Self. This is very precious. Sometimes, you may feel bored. It does not matter. Just be aware that you are burning some old seeds of boredom. If you are averse to boredom, the boredom will never leave you. If you are bored with yourself, just think how boring you would be to somebody else? So even if you are bored, never mind. It will make you more and more sensitive. Know that you are just burning something – *tapas*. You should think that it is a *tapas*, and that you are doing penance. You should willingly just take the step and be determined to do it, however boring it is. You often take up challenges with friends. Similarly, take up this challenge. To get over your boredom, kindle the challenge in you.

Chapter 9

ELIMINATING THE CAUSE OF PAIN

If you just look into all the pleasures or joy that you get in life, you will note that they all come with a tax and this tax is sorrow.

In the next sutra, Patanjali says,

परिणामतापसंस्कार दुः खैर्गुणवृत्तिविरोधाश्च दुः खमेव सर्व विवेकिनः

Parinaama taapa sanskaara dukhaihi guna vrittivirodhaascha dukhameva sarvam vivekinah.

Every event causes some pain. An event could be very pleasant and joyful. But, it comes with a little pinch, a pain. The pain is that, however joyful an event is, it will end. And the ending of an event, however pleasurable and joyful, comes with a little pinch. The greater the joy it has given, the greater will be the pain when it ends.

Parinaama dukha - This is called *parinaama*, the effect or the result.

Taapa dukha – longing for an event. Waiting for a pleasurable event causes pain.

Samskaara dukha – the impressions of it, memories of it. Memories of a pleasure also bring pain. So before you have something, the feverishness to get it is painful. Then, when you have it, the fear of losing it is painful. And, when it is gone the memory of its joy is painful. So the whole thing is all pain from the beginning to the end.

A *viveki* or an intelligent person whose wisdom has been awakened sees the whole thing as a pain. So there is nothing that is not pain. *Sarvam eva dukha mayam.* Everything is painful. You say love is so beautiful, but love is also painful. How close can you get to the person you love? Bodies get close but still there is no satisfaction. Each one wants to enter the other's body. How can it enter? How much it can enter? You get frustrated. Often, in the next life, a male takes up a female body and a female takes up a male body. This is because it is the most prominent craving, or longing in the mind. A male longs for a female and a female longs for a male. This is also the reason that in every male there will be female characteristics and, likewise, in a female, on account of some impressions of the previous birth.

The soul is not satisfied with the physical body coming close. It wants something more. It wants to merge. It wants to vanish and disappear. This is what is called love. In love, there are two expressions – the first is that one wants to disappear into the other, and the other is that one wants to eat the other so that he/she disappears. These are the two expressions that lovers say to each other. They do not know why they are saying. They are not cannibals! Does love make you a cannibal! Really, if that was possible, each one would do it, literally – gulp down their boyfriends or girlfriends. Then, there would be no more worry. They would not have to be bothered about who they are looking at and where they are going. Otherwise, the mind would be constantly engaged in checking. Lovers become watchdogs after a while. Often when they come to the course, they do not meditate. Their attention is ever on their boyfriends or girlfriends. And they have to be told to meditate without any worries; that, their boyfriends or girlfriends would be taken care of.

Love creates pain; a tremendous amount of pain and so does separation. A wish creates much pain and pressurizes the mind. And then trying to please somebody creates pain, and to know whether they are pleased or not pleased also creates pain. You want to totally know the mind of the other person. How is this possible? You do not even know your own mind. So, how can you know somebody else's mind? And it is impossible to know anybody's mind just by their words. They say the tongue has no bone, so it can just move in any way it wants. It has no value; no loyalty. It is not steady. It may say something one day and something totally opposite the next. You cannot trust your tongue even if you can trust anything in the world.

You feel good and joyful when you do what somebody else

wishes. However, suddenly this feeling is not there. Now, doing what had given you joy becomes painful. It needs an effort to do spiritual practices and that is painful. If you don't do it, it is more painful. One day, you may not be feeling good and you attribute it to your not having meditated that day. Or, after you have meditated, you feel you have not done it long enough. And that is the reason you are not getting the good effects. You find something to complain about.

Sarvam evam dukham mayam. If you really look with the eyes of wisdom, you will find that there is not a bit in this creation, which is devoid of pain. Pain is the tail which comes along with everything in the world. If you do something, you will get a free coupon of pain with it.

The next sutra is about what you will do then? When you realize that everything is pain, then how do you go about? What do you do? You have to do something to stop this pain. What will you do?

हेयं दु:खमनागतम्

Heyam dukham anaagatam.

The root cause of pain needs to be eliminated. That pain which has not yet come in life and that sorrow which has not yet sprouted should be nipped right in the beginning. How do we do that?

द्रष्टदृश्योः संयोगो हेयहेतुः

Drashta drishyayoh sanyogo heyahetuh.

The main cause of pain is forgetting that one's Self is separate from one's environment. The Self, the seer and the seen - lack of perception of the Self and the objects that are all around the Self. You think of yourself as you. Then the problems begin. Usually, we keep our life somewhere else and not in us.

There was a story in the olden days.

The life of the king was in a parrot. So, if this parrot was killed, the king would die, too. The king's life was not in the king. He would not die if somebody did anything to him. He was like a superman. If the King had to be killed, the assassin had to go to a remote island which had a fort. It was very difficult to get into it. If the assassin did manage to get in, he had to enter a palace inside the fort. The palace was full of cobras. He had to get past them. Then, he had to go underground where a door would open. Inside would be a cage with a parrot in it. However, the assassin could not touch the cage. If he did, it would burn him down. The parrot had to be killed without touching the cage. Only then would the king die.

This life is not in one's Self. That life is somewhere else; in a bank account. You have not just deposited money in the bank.

You have deposited your life, too. You will die if the bank closes or if something else happens to it. When you give something more important than life, then that becomes the cause of your suffering. You can experience that you are not the body through meditation. You can see the difference between the surroundings and the seer, the light.

That is what Patanjali says,

प्रकाशक्रियास्थितिशीलं भूतेन्द्रियात्मकं भोगापवर्गार्थं दृश्यम्

Prakaasha kriya sthitisheelam bhootendriyaatmakam bhoga apavargaartha drishyam.

This does not mean that you have to run away from this world. This world is here for your enjoyment. Patanjali was very clear about it. The beautiful sceneries are there for you to look at. The good food is there for you to eat and enjoy. The whole world is here for you to enjoy, but while enjoying do not forget your Self. You are separate from them. This is *viveka*.

प्रकाशक्रियास्थितिशीलं भूतेन्द्रियात्मकं भोगापवर्गार्थं दृश्यम्

Prakaasha kriya sthitisheelam bhootendriyaatmakam bhoga apavargaartha drishyam.

The world which is seen is illuminated. Each thing gives you a message. It gives you an idea of how great the consciousness is. Every aspect in this world is an expression of consciousness and everything is active.

Prakaasha means manifesting. Everything has manifested out of consciousness. *Kriya* - everything in this universe is dynamic. They are not static. Flowers come up. The mountains appear to be static but they are not. They are all dynamic. Every atom in this universe is dynamic.

Sthiti means everything undergoes certain stages of evolution. Everything has a stage, a state. And everything is governed by certain principles and qualities.

Bhootendriyaatmakam. The entire creation is made up of five elements - the five elements and five sense organs. There are five organs of perception and five organs of action. These are ten organs. The entire creation is endowed with these ten and the mind.

Bhoga apavargaartham. This entire creation is there to give you pleasure and relief. Whatever gives you pleasure should also give you relief. Otherwise, the pleasure becomes a pain. You may like *gulab jamun.* You can have one, two, three or four; then, maybe, the fifth one, becomes a little too much. And then the more you have, the greater is your discomfort. Something that gave you pleasure is now making you suffer.

If you are forced to eat twenty apple-pies you will hold your head, and pray that you want relief from it and want to get away from them. It is the same with music. For how long can you enjoy music? One hour, two hours, or three hours if someone forces you. If you have to hear music for twenty-four hours a day and seven days a week, you will appeal to be relieved of listening to it. The wonderful music, which gave you so much pleasure, causes pain if the listening is overdone. So that has to give you a relief also.

The entire creation does give you enjoyment and liberation. You have to get yourself liberated from all these at some time or other. Otherwise, they will become a pain; the pleasure will become a pain.

Then, Patanjali went on to describe the grades in this. They are *sattvic, rajasic,* and *tamasic. Tamasic* things bring more dullness. *Rajasic* brings greater activity and *Sattvic* more light, and freedom. If you take wholesome food, it is good for your health and gives you pleasure. But if you take drugs, they entrap you. They seem to be give pleasure to begin with but gives you only pain and suffering. And they are hard to get out of. So drugs are *tamasic.*

Sattvic, tamasic, rajasic. The three grades; the whole creation is made up of these three *gunas,* three natures. Some foods make you duller and some more agitated. Everything arises from these three *gunas.* There are some specialities about each. The creation is made up of so many details.

द्रष्टा दृशिमात्रः शुद्धोऽपि प्रत्ययानुपश्यः

Drishtaa drishi maatrah shuddho api pratyaya anupashyah.

The Self, though it is ever pure and untainted, is just a witness. However, when it becomes one with the *buddhi*, the intellect, then it gets coloured. It seems coloured. It seems just like somebody who, stuck in their own intellect, continues to be with their thoughts and ideas, as though they are their own. They suffer a lot as a result of this. The Self is the centre of the whole creation.

The next sutra says,

तदर्थ एव दृश्यस्यात्मा

Tadartha eva drishyasyaatma.

Though this world does not exist for the one who is realized and enlightened the way it does for the enlightened, it continues to exist with its opposites. There is no more suffering for the one who is awakened in knowledge. The world appears completely different and all of this creation is filled with bliss, or part of the Self. But, for the others, it exists as they see it. So, you may not be considering this world separate from your Self, but as a part of your Self. It does not exist for you, but for others it does exist. It is just like your leaving a plane or a bus after a journey. For you the journey is over. But the plane or bus keeps going on. They need to takes others onwards. The bus does not stop just because your journey is over.

कृतार्थं प्रति नष्टमप्यनष्टं तदन्यसाधारणत्वात्

Kritaartham   prati   nashtam   anashtam   tadanya
saadhaaranatvaat.

There is a power of nature in these *sutras* and we should really go deep into them. Your body is made up of the three *gunas* – *sattva, rajas* and *tamas,* and they influence your thoughts, behavioural patterns, etc. Many things may happen in the world and the *gunas* attract, accordingly, the events, situations and circumstances around you. When the *tamasic guna* dominates, it creates more dullness, sleep, and lethargy in you. When the *rajasic guna* is dominating, your mind is restless and full of desires. And if the mind is dominated by *sattva guna,* it is very alert, sharp, joyful and enthusiastic. All these qualities emerge. Now, when these three *gunas* influence you, according to their nature, time, place, etc., you tend to identify yourself with the effect of that influence. You may begin to feel that you are a dull and lethargic person; that you have many negative qualities. This is ignorance. You should observe the tendencies that come up in you and think you are not those tendencies; that the *gunas* will influence you according to their nature.

There is another story. There was a very great monk, who lived in the Himalayas. He had free access to all the places because the people loved him and welcomed him. He would have lunch at the King's palace everyday. The Queen would serve him lunch in a golden plate and cup. He would just eat go away. This was a routine. When he left one day he took a silver glass and a golden spoon without telling anybody. The Queen and the other people in the palace noticed this. They wondered why he had done it. And he had not told anybody, either. He had just put them in his bag and had left. Three days later, he brought the items back. This was even more puzzling. Earlier, they had thought that, maybe he had needed them and had taken them. But his returning them was even more puzzling.

So the King called all the wise people of the kingdom. He asked them the reason for the monk's behaviour. They asked the King to check what food had been given to the monk on the previous couple of days. It was discovered that the food had been cooked with grains and provisions confiscated from some robbers who had been arrested some days back. Eating that food had awakened the tendency to rob in him and had made him steal the objects.

In ancient days people gave much important to these points. If somebody did something unusual, they would go to the root cause for it. So, instead of accusing the monk of stealing, they found out what made him do it – the root cause.

तस्य हेतुरविद्या

Tasya heturavidyaa.

If you think these *vrittis* are yours, it is ignorance. And what is the way to come out of the ignorance - a definite understanding and knowledge in the mind that the body is undergoing changes all the time; that the world is undergoing changes all the time; that the entire universe, in the form of fluids, is in a state of fluidity - it is all full of changes and is going on, on its own, according to its nature.

The definite knowledge that you are not the body, that you are the Self, that you are the space, that you are imperishable, untouched and untamed by the *prakriti* and the world around you, that the body is all hollow and empty, and every particle in this body is ever changing, and that the mind is ever changing is the way to get out of this cycle.

Chapter 10

THE EIGHT LIMBS OF YOGA

Human consciousness is like a seed. A seed has the possibility of a tree, of branches, of leaves, flowers and fruits, of multiplication, etc. So does the human mind. A seed needs a proper soil, proper conditions, sunlight and water to sprout and blossom in its possibility. It is the same with the human consciousness, the human mind.

Either the seed can be dormant for many years, keeping its sprouting and developing possibilities within itself or it can start sprouting and growing right away. The sprouting of this seed of human consciousness is *viveka* – discrimination and wisdom. Freedom comes with *viveka,* or discrimination. All other species in this creation are completely governed by nature. They do not need discrimination nor do they have freedom. So they never break the laws of nature. The human consciousness and the human mind have been given this freedom. So, it has also been given discrimination. It is through this *viveka*, wisdom and discrimination, that a human consciousness and human mind, can be governed to progress or to remain where it is. Generally, you will not find any animal overeating if it is sick. It may do this only if it is mad. Normally animals eat in time. They rest in time and mate in time. They have no choice. But human beings have the freedom to do whatever they want. This freedom is given along with discrimination, with wisdom, with the consequences of action and with knowledge of consequences of action. This is to enable humans to choose and lead a life of wisdom.

The speciality of human life is that it is governed by *viveka* – wisdom and discrimination. And how can this be enhanced? How can this seed be made to sprout and grow into a sapling? Then it needs watering again and again, until it grows. A seed has the possibility, but if it is not watered then the possibility remains a possibility, and does not manifest.

Here Patanjali steps in and says,

Yogaangaanushtaana – the seed may be sprouted and made to grow by practicing and observing the limbs of Yoga. Through Yoga, *ashuddhikshaye,* the impurities get eliminated, *aa viveka khyaatehe* – the *viveka*, the wisdom, shines forth. The husk is gone and the sprout comes up.

Now, what are the limbs of Yoga?

Patanjali said that there were eight limbs of Yoga. They were *Yama, niyama, aasana, pranayama, pratyahara, dharana, dhyana* and *samaadhi.*

He went into the details of each and the results to be expected from it. Yoga has eight limbs, just as a chair has four legs. Each is connected to the whole. So, if you just pull one, the whole chair will move. The whole body develops together. Organs develop together. It is not that the nose develops first, and then the ears. That is why Patanjali called them the limbs of Yoga. Unfortunately, people think that these are stages and come one after the other; that we have to achieve each, one by one. This is not right. It is a misconception.

Yama is the first limb. What are *yamas*? *Ahimsa satya asteya brahmacharya aparigraha.* There are five *yamas*.

Ahimsa – non-violence, *satya* – truth, *asteya* – non-stealing, *brahmacharya* – moving in Brahman, moving in the bigness, *aparigraha* – non-accumulation.

जातिदेशकालसमयनवश्चिन्हसर्वभुममहाव्रतम्

Jaati desha kaala samaya nvachchinnaaha saarvabhoumaa mahaavratam.

These are the greatest vows because it is applicable at all times, in all places and for all people. There are certain laws which apply just to certain people, places, or times. An animal is violent for some reason. The wild animals hunt only when they are hungry. They do not hunt just for pleasure but the human beings do. They go hunting for no reason. A python eats one rat a month and sleeps for the rest of the month. Just one rat a month is good enough for it though it is scary and dangerous. If it swallows a goat or eats something bigger, it will not harm or kill any animal for several months. But human beings in the name of God, in the name of love, kill each other. In this world, mindless violence is prevalent in the name of country, religion, etc. This is total lack of *viveka*, wisdom. A violent man cannot hear anybody. His ears are sealed.

Violence is the result of frustrations. The mind gets frustrated. The frustration builds up. A big question mark may come up. And that very question turns into violence. And it catches on to the surroundings. A crowd may become violent. Individually a person may not be able to do a violent act. However, in a crowd, he will join hands with everybody and be violent.

Viveka can dawn when a person takes this vow of non-violence – that he will not kill or take any life on this planet consciously. Unconsciously, you may be destroying many creatures when you walk. You may be stepping on and killing may small creatures like ants. But you are not killing them consciously. It is happening. But an intention to destroy something or to be violent can cut your own roots. Dropping this intention for violence is *ahimsa*.

And then *satya* – to be with what is right now, to be with something that is non-changing. To know that something, deep in you, is non-changing. *Satya* does not mean just speaking truth. *Satya* is total commitment to the truth. It is not just with words. Unfortunately, people mistake *satya* to mean just speaking the truth.

What is the effect of *ahimsa?*

अहिंसाप्रतिष्ठायां तत्सन्निधौ वैरत्यागः

Ahimsa pratishtaayaam tat sannidhau vairatyaagah.

If you are established in non-violence, violence will be dropped in your very presence by other creatures. Someone may plan to attack you. But, as soon as they come near you, they will feel your vibration which is totally non-violent. Then, they will stop being violent.

The contemporary of Buddha was Mahaveera. He was the promoter of the Jain religion. He emphasized *ahimsa*. It is said that people up to twenty kilometres around him would drop their violence. And, that, even thorns would not prick anybody. They would become soft and be flat on the ground to avoid pricking anybody.

अहिंसाप्रतिष्ठायां तत्सन्निधौ वैरत्यागः

Ahimsa pratishtaayaam tat sannidhau vairatyaagah.

If you are established in non-violence, other creatures will drop violence in your presence.

सत्यप्रतिष्ठायां क्रियाफलाश्रयत्वम्

Satya pratishthaayaam kriyaphalaashrayatvam.

All your actions will become fruitful, if you are established in truth. The actions of many people do not bring about results because there is no truth-consciousness in them. The fruit of an action will follow immediately when there is no truth-consciousness.

Kriyaphalaashrayatvam – There is success in action. And truth is not just the words. It is the quality of the consciousness, of straight-forwardness. Even if you are telling a lie and you are bold enough to say that you are telling a lie then you are speaking truth.

When you tell a lie, your consciousness is not solid. It is not straight-forward. There is no strength in it.

Satya pratishtaayaam kriyaphalaashrayatvam. Success comes easily to a person who is committed to truth; who is committed to "what is"- the presence of being. It is not that he will not encounter failures. He may encounter failure, but he will win. *Satyameva jayate*, is a slogan, like, "We trust in God" which is written on the American currency notes. In India, the slogan is "The truth alone triumphs". Truth will definitely win, though intermittently, it may appear not to be winning.

There is a story. At one time, India was a collection of many small kingdoms. They were ruled by an Emperor. Akbar, a

Mughal emperor had a wise minister called Birbal. He was very humorous. The Emperor would pass odd laws and rules. Once he ordered that anybody found telling a lie would be hanged. At that time the emperors and kings could make their own laws, any laws that they fancied. There was no parliament or congressmen to debate and pass laws. He heard a talk on truth and had been influenced. His new law created a big commotion. The lawyers felt that it would ruin their business and their profession would be finished. They had a meeting to decide the course of action.

Similarly, all the merchants gathered for a meeting to discuss the new law. They wondered how they would be able to sell their products. It was disastrous. Despite being aware that their products were not the best, they would claim them to be so. They would tell many lies to their potential customers and employ various gimmicks of business. With the new law, they would be ruined. They felt that it was outrageous. That they would not be able to carry on with the new law in place. There were similar meetings held by the astrologers, priests, doctors, etc.

They approached Birbal, a wise minister in the King's court. They requested him to do something. He promised that he would. The next day Birbal went to the King's bedroom. The guards outside stopped him. He told them that he was going to get hanged. It was a lie because the king's room was not a place where he would be hanged. So the guards took him to the King. If he was hanged, then he didn't speak a lie; whatever he said was truth. Then the King would have punished an innocent man. And that would be a big crime that the King would commit. If King did not hang him, then the law would have become obsolete.

To settle this, the King called all the ministers and pundits and there was a big debate. If Birbal was hanged, a law would be violated him and if he was not hanged, then, too, a law would be violated. The King was in a fix, and everybody was in a greater fix. Finally, they asked Birbal to suggest what was to be done.

Birbal said that truth is not what is spoken. Anything that is spoken becomes a lie. The moment you say something, you are distorting "what is" and "what is" is truth."

Following *satya* is to be with "what is." To be truthful in one's life, one's presence, one's mind, one's heart – not in your words but in your intention. Are your intentions straight-forward and clear? Or are you hiding something behind them? Is there some other hook you are keeping? That indicates the truth. The second principle, *yama*, is the clarity in your intention and openness in your approach, the truth.

Third *yama,* is *asteya,* not stealing. You may admire somebody's voice and wish you had a good one. You have already stolen it. You may admire someone's looks and wish you looked like her. You have already stolen her looks. This creates jealousy and a desire to have something that you admire. This is the reason why people steal. *Asteya* eliminates jealousy and the tendency to steal. People steal many things. Some people steal someone else's plans, others steal techniques. Then, again, someone steals other's things. These things do not work. People who steal remain poor.

If you are committed to be sincere and do not steal, then *sarva ratnopalabdihi* – all the wealth comes to you effortlessly. This is the effect of not stealing. A little intention to steal can keep you poor. Most of the time poverty is self-induced. A person wants to be sneaky and try to grab as much as he can. That is where his luck goes down the drain. Not stealing brings all the wealth.

ब्रम्हचर्यप्रतिष्ठायां वीर्यलाभः

Bramhacharya pratishtaayaam veeryalaabhah.

Brahmacharya, usually means celibacy. Celibacy brings you a lot of strength. *Brahmacharya* has a bigger and deeper meaning than just celibacy. *Brahma* means infinity, *charya* means moving in the infinity. You move like a glow of light when you know your vast nature and consider yourself not to be just the body. This is when celibacy naturally happens. When you are sitting in deep meditation, you do not feel you are a body and that you are a lump of heavy weight – eighty pounds, ninety pounds, one hundred pound body. You feel so light. You feel as though you are like a feather. When you walk you do not feel the weight of your body. You feel more space. The more joyful you are, the less do you feel the body. The more you are in infinite consciousness, the lesser will you feel the tension, or the physical bodily weight, or presence. That is *brahmacharya*. Our consciousness expanded to the infinite and moving in the infinity is our true nature.

The nature that is space brings a lot of vigour, valour and strength in you. A person, may be ever small-minded and looking around to check who is good looking or with whom he or she can have sex. Such persons will have low energy and will be very dull and nobody will go near them. A person who is obsessed with sex is unattractive. And they create such a thick and dull vibration around them that there is no strength, vigour or commitment in them. Nothing comes out of them. They can be seen in places like bars. They have no strength at all. They just go anywhere and after anybody without even knowing where they are going.

There is a story about Mullah Nasseruddin. Mullah Nasseruddin was watching a dance on a movie screen. The actress was dancing, and Mullah was watching the dance, waiting and waiting. Suddenly Mullah went flat on the floor. His wife asked what he was looking at. He replied that he wanted to see the dance of the lady more closely. That, he was waiting for her to sit down.

The mind becomes so crazy that there is no strength in it. It gets to be limited and then jealousy, anger, irritation and frustration raise their heads. And when these storms of negativity arise in a mind, it becomes very weak and poor. All the truth about existence disappears. When your mind is obsessed with such a load of negativity, you cannot even observe the beautiful nature that you are in.

Brahmacharya pratishtaayaam veeryalaabhaha. Great strength comes when *Brahmacharya* is established in one. That is when you consider yourself more than just the body. You see yourself as consciousness, as *Brahma.*

अपरिग्रहस्तेय जन्मकथायांतासम्बोध:

Aparigrahasthaiye janmakathayanta sambodhaha.

When you do not accumulate then you get knowledge of previous births and knowledge of different species. The communication in you improves. When a person wants more and more, he just thinks of himself and is obsessed with fear. He does not know the eternal value of life. Life has been there from ages and will continue for ages to come. Non-accumulation means confidence in one's existence and in one's ability, and having knowledge of one's self. If you know how to make bread, then you will not go on making bread for a week and then store it for a year in your room. It will become stale and inedible.

In China, there is a proverb, "What you give, you gain more.

Whatever you scatter, you will have it all. You lose what you hold on to." When you scatter, it all comes back to you. Everything is yours and you are all over. A person who is very afraid of himself and who has no idea of his strength is very stingy. A person who is very selfish and stingy stores and stores; he accumulates.

A very wealthy gentleman was dying. He was on his death bed. However, he was on the phone checking the prices on the share market. He was going to die at any moment but he was concerned about the share prices and how much he was gaining and how much he was losing. But, he would have to leave everything after death. If money transfer was possible to the other side of death, people would transfer all their assets before dying. Lawyers would not have to write wills. Fortunately or unfortunately, this is not possible. People accumulate and accumulate, and then they die. This does not mean that we should not save money. But Patanjali has asked what the effect of it was?

Janmakathayanta sambodhaha. When you give things to people, it brings back something to you. There are some good vibrations and this makes you happy. If you are very unhappy one day, then give away something or give some gifts to somebody. Then, your consciousness will change, shift. And sometimes when you accept gifts from someone, you will feel unhappy. In the ancient days, they knew this science very well. They used to call wise people to their homes and give them food and gifts.

And, when they accepted, they would give one more offering. This was to show thankfulness to the wise people for having accepted their offering. This was called *dakshina*.

So, if someone accepts a gift, then the giver should be thankful. This is called *dakshina*. The giver is thankful because they are not just taking something. The acceptors are giving back their mind and taking away certain impressions or *karmas* of the past from the giver's mind. Non-acceptance or non-accumulation of objects, or things from people, is *asteya*.

Parigraha is always receiving and wondering what will be received. If you do not accept anything from anybody, you will feel different. This is practically not possible in the world. There are people who practice this to the extreme. You do not have to go to the extreme but being aware of this fact is useful.

These are the five *mahavratas* – the great rules, the great vows. You will get results according to the extent of your practice.

विपक्षभादने प्रतिपक्षभवानम्

Vipakshabhadane pratipaksha bhavaanam.

Suppose your mind feels that you do not care about the rules. That you want to do what you wish to. If you wish to be violent, you will be so.

To counter this Patanjali said *vipakshabhadane pratipaksha bhavaanam* – to do the opposite.

Before mentioning this, he also mentioned the *niyamas*. What are the *niyamas*?

There are the five *yamas*, and then the five *niyamas*.

The *niyamas* are,

शौचसन्तोषतपः स्वाध्यायेश्वरप्रणिधानानि नियमाः

Shaucha santosha tapaha swaadhyaaya eshwara pranidhaanaani niyamaah.

Shaucha is physical purity; keeping oneself clean. People may not take a bath for several days and wear perfumes. This is not cleanliness. Water should run in and on this body -both inside and outside. You have to drink enough water and let it run through your system. Water is the greatest purifier for this physical body. There needs to be cleanliness in the atmosphere and in the environment. If you are used to being unclean, you do not feel anything if you are. You can see this in the slums. The people there do not mind living in very dirty conditions, with garbage all around. It just does not register in their consciousness. They are used to it. In the same way, you get used to being unclean, and keeping your room unclean, etc. It starts with your postponing your bath one day or wearing the clothes that you wore the previous day. And then, something or the other comes up and you are very busy for a few days and do not have the time to take a bath. You are not aware of the foul smell emanating from you but somebody else will be bothered by it. And it is worse if you use perfumes. You will not be aware of your odour for very long. Regular bathing and keeping personal hygiene is very essential. And mind also needs to be kept clean – *antaha shaucha* – *bahya bheetara shaucha*. It needs outer cleanliness, inner cleanliness and freedom from tension.

Santosha – contentment and happiness. Happiness is an attitude. If you are used to being unhappy, you will grumble and be unhappy even in the best of situations. Nothing can make you happy in the world. What happens when you are happy; when you smile? There is much relaxation on your face - in the muscles of the face, in the head, etc. There is freedom, joy and relaxation. And if you have trained your muscles and your nervous system to be unhappy, then there will be knots and stresses on your face. There will be stiffness in your head and in your body and you will remain unhappy irrespective of the situation, surrounding, etc. *Santosha* is a practice. Being happy is a practice. Unconditional happiness is a practice. You need to decide that you are going to smile, no matter what happens. You need to feel that everyone and everything is going to die and disappear, anyway. So, you do not care. You need to feel that you will be happy, smile and, at least, enjoy your breath. And that you will not mind if somebody else is upset and something else is wrong. At least you can breathe happily. Nobody is going to hold your nose. If you will feel like this, then you are free.

You sell your happiness for peanuts. You sell your smile for a penny. The entire world is not worth your smile. Even if you are made a King or an Emperor of the world, it is not worth giving away your smile. This is *niyama* – the rule, the condition for Yoga.

One of the limbs is *Santosha* – being happy. What could make you unhappy? Losing a lot of money? Could that make you unhappy? So what! Anyway, you are going to lose this body, which is going to enjoy those millions of dollars. It has to happen. So many people had millions of dollars and they died. What else are you unhappy about? Is your friend leaving you? Your own body is going to desert you. Why are you so worried about your friend deserting you? Sometimes people lose things one by one and sometimes they lose everything together. This is the only chance. Either you lose everything at one time, or you keep losing them one by one. So when you lose your friend, you should think that you may have lost one friend. And, that the body is going to be lost after sometime. So, it does not matter.

Consider yourself to be in the second category - losing things one by one. You are not going to die along with your friend, or you are not going to take them to heaven, even if they don't want to come. Everyone has his own ticket, time and place booked. There you cannot make any demands. So, why not be happy now? The strength of your happiness is measured by your adverse situations. If everything is smooth then your big smile is worth nothing. You should smile in any adverse situation. You should feel that, even if the world dies and disappears, you are not going to sell your smile and that you are not going to be unhappy. This strength in you is *santosha*. This is an attitude you develop.

There is another Mullah Nasseruddin story.

Mullah Nasseruddin would grumble all the time. He was a farmer. So, he would grumble that there were no rains because of which no crops were growing. It was all so difficult. However, that year there was very good rainfall and he had good crops in his field. People thought that Nasseruddin would not grumble because the crops were good and he would be happy. However, when they went to congratulate him for his good crops, Mullah had his usual long face. He said that, with the good crops he had so much work to do. All the previous years he did not have to do anything since there were no crops. But, with the good crops, he would have to go to market to sell them. It was a big headache. So, whether Mullah had crops or not, his grumbling continued.

It is the same in your life. You are unhappy about the things you have and you are unhappy, too, about those that you don't have. Someone who does not have a car is unhappy, because he does not have one. And when he buys one, is unhappy, because he has to maintain it and pay the tax. It is all such a big headache. He feels that, earlier, he just needed to take a public transport and go wherever he wanted to. Now he has to have his car serviced regularly. And, when he goes out, he has to hunt around for a parking space for it.

Santosha is developing the habit of being happy. You have to develop it yourself. Nobody else can do it for you. Nothing else can give it to you. If anybody else or anything else gives it, it will only be temporary. You should adopt *santosha* as your rule in life.

Shaucha and *santhosha* - cleanliness and happiness.

Tapaha, swadhyaaya, ishwara pranidhana – You need to have some *tapas* - endurance and patience, *Swadhyaaya* – self-study and *ishwara pranidhana* - devotion to God, to the Lord.

These are the five rules.

विपक्षभादने प्रतिपक्षभवानम्

vipakshabhadane pratipaksha bhavaanam.

When the opposite of these bothers you and when your mind rebels against these principles and rules, then you should bring up the feelings, which are the opposite. And what are those?

Patanjali says,

वितर्का हिंसादयः कृतकारितानुमोदिता लोभक्रोधमोहपूर्वका मृदुमध्याधिमात्रा
दुःखाज्ञानानन्तफला इति प्रतिपक्षभावनम्

Vitarka hinsaadayah krita karita anumoditaa lobha krodha moha purvakaa mridu madhya adhimatra duhkhagyanaan anantyaphalaa iti pratipaksha bhaavanam.

There are three types of violence, untruth and all the opposite values. These can be done by us or we can make somebody else do them because we do not want to do it ourselves or we can agree with somebody who does it. They arise from *lobha* – greed, *krodha* – anger and *moha* – delusion. When you are greedy, you make someone else do what you want to be done. The negative principles thrive because of greed, violence, or untruth. When a person is greedy, he does not see things as they are. This is also true of a person who is angry. His discriminating mind gets clouded and he loses his powers of discrimination. He is not aware of what he is doing.

So, when you do something or approve of some action, you should check if it is anger, attachment or your delusions which is stimulating you. They could be mild, medium or in excess.

They bring sorrow, *dukha* and *ajnaana,* ignorance - a chain of sorrow and ignorance. This is what the opposite values do. When you are aware of this, you may avoid them and adhere to your rules.

There are millions of people out there in the world who are engaged in violent activities. You may wonder why they are doing it. It is because they are not aware that such activities will bring them more suffering, pain and ignorance. Suffering is not palatable. It is not pleasing to anybody in the world. Even a cockroach does not want to suffer, not even an ant. Despite this fact that no human being wants to suffer, why are so many people engaged in criminal activity? Patanjali said that we should wake up and be aware of this.

शौचात् स्वागंजुगुप्सा परैंसंसर्गः

Shouchat svaanga jugupsa paraih sansargah.

With personal hygiene and cleanliness, your attachment to the physical body is lifted up. You become more aware of your inner Self – the light and inner body that you are.

Svaanga jugupsa – craving for certain parts of the body begins in our mind, because one does not understand this body totally. Underneath this skin, it is all bones, flesh, nerves, etc. This lack of total understanding of the body brings up different forms of obsessions and mania in people. They cannot be satisfied with anything but their obsessions. And, they become violent. That is why there are many crimes related to the body. People kill just for fun. So many crimes of sex are committed. It is lack of understanding of one's own body.

Shaucha, cleanliness establishes *sattva shuddhi* - the mind becomes *sattvic*; the brain, the *buddhi* and the intellect gets purified. *Saumanasya* – the mind becomes even and harmonious. There is *Ekaagrata* – one-pointedness and *indriya jayatva* – control over one's sense organs. Then, *aatma darshana yogyatvaani cha* – the ability to realize one's Self comes to you because of this purity. When you are very unhappy or depressed, you avoid being in contact with anybody. This is natural. It is inbuilt in our system. At such times, you want to be away from everybody and just be by yourself. This is very natural. Not being in contact with anybody can bring about a certain amount of purity in you. It can awaken the ability to realize yourself. It can make your brain and mind more one-pointed. It can bring clarity in thinking. That is why most of the great works in the world have come up in solitude. A person has to be alone to write a great poem. A great painter wants to be alone when he wants to paint something.

However, sometimes people take this to extremes. They feel that having no contact means not even being touched. People shy away from others. This science has been misused, in various ways. But this is a truth. If you do not touch anybody or are not be in contact with anybody for a day or two, your mind will get back to its shape. These are the effects of *shaucha.*

संन्तोषादनुत्तमः सुखलाभः

Santoshaad anuttamah sukha laabhah.

Santosha is happiness and contentment which gives great joy. *Anuttama*, the greatest happiness can be got by just cultivating this habit and this attitude of being happy. It will, in turn, destroy your misery. It is not just a mood-lifting process. It is an attitude. You develop this attitude to be happy. And it will bring you the greatest happiness - an incomparable happiness in life.

कायेन्द्रियसिद्धिरशुद्धिक्षयात् तपसः

Kaayendriya siddhih ashuddhi kshyaat tapasah.

The body and the senses become *strong* with *tapas*. When you fast, you are not pleasing God. You are not ensuring your enlightenment or a passage to heaven. When you fast and do various practices, your body becomes strong. It can withstand great heat and cold. Your resistance power increases. *Ashuddhi kshyaa* –the impurities are eliminated.

स्वाध्यायादिष्टदेवतासम्प्रयोगः

Swadhyaaya dishta devata samprayogah.

By self-study, *swadhyaaya*, the *devas* or divine presence is felt and experienced. By self-study, by observing and by being hollow and empty, you become a channel. You become a part of the divine. You are able to feel the presence of divinity. The angels and *devas*, which are different forms of your consciousness, start blossoming.

समाधिसिद्धिरीश्वरप्रणिधानात्

Samaadhi siddhih ishvara pranidhaanaat.

Samadhi comes about by one-pointed devotion to the divine.

स्थिरसुखमासनम्

Sthira sukham aasanam.

Patanjali mentioned all the *yamas* and *niyamas*.

Now what is *asana*? *Sthira sukham asanam* – Asana is that which is steady and comfortable. Normally, when you are comfortable, you are not steady. You will not be sitting erect. But when you are erect, you will be so stiff that you will not be comfortable. But when you are in *asana*, you are erect, steady and at the same time comfortable. *Sthira sukham asanam.*

And what is the effect of *asana*?

प्रयत्नशैथिल्यानन्तसमापत्तिभ्याम्

Prayatna shaithilya ananta samaapattibhyaam.

Prayatna shaithilya – letting go the effort. The main point of this is feeling the body, letting go of the effort and experiencing the infinity - harmonizing oneself with the infinity. We do this while doing *asanas*. Have you noticed that when you do *asanas* with total awareness, you feel totally spaced out later. *Prayatna shaithilya* is to let go of the effort and sit in a comfortable posture - *sukham asanam* pleasurable. You feel that it is a pleasure just to be; just to sit. This is *sukha*. *Sukha* means pleasure. Have you ever sat steadily feeling that it is wonderful just to be; just to sit? If you do it once, you will see how it feels. *Prayatna shaithilya* is letting go of all the effort and feeling the infinity.

What is the effect of this? What does it do?

ततो द्वन्द्वानभिघातः

Tato dwandwa anabhighaatah.

It strikes at the duality or the conflicts in you. It roots them out.

Dwanda anabhighaataha. You should do *asana* whenever you are confused and your mind is in conflict. Sit in an *asana* and there will be clarity right away. The effect of an *asana* is clearing out all conflicts and dualities.

तस्मिन् सति श्वासप्रश्वासयोर्गतिविच्छेदः प्राणायामः

Tasmin sati shwaasa prashwaasa yogah gati vichchhedah pranayamah.

It is natural to obstruct the flow of breath in an *asana*.. Patanjali said that it is obstructing the natural flow of your breath because it is not natural at all. You have made your breath very unnatural. So whatever you feel is natural, is not actually natural. We have to return to the natural way of breathing. We do this by *gati vichchedaha* – breaking its movement. We break its movement consciously by breathing deep, long and subtle, with counts and by keeping our attention on different parts of the body. That is the next *sutra*.

Baahya abhyantara stambha vritti desha kaala sankhya bhih paridrishtau deergha sukshmaha.

In just one *sutra*, Patanjali has described all the *pranayamas*.

Breathe in, hold, breathe out, and hold – with different counts and with attention on various parts of the body. That is all. Most of the *pranayamas* are there in one sentence; in one sutra.

Baahya abhyantara vishaya akshepi chaturtaha.

But there is one more *pranayama*, which happens automatically. When all the thoughts and ideas are cleared from the mind, there is a natural *pranayama*. It throws out all the impurities from the mind. That is the fourth *pranayama*.

Baahya abhyantara vishaya akshepi chaturtaha.

Patanjali said that *pranayama* should be learnt with proper guidance. It is not to be done on one's own and anywhere. The *pranayama* which happens all by itself and without any effort is the fourth *pranayama*. You go deep and the *pranayama* starts. It breaks the routine way of breathing. It assumes or forms its own rhythm. This is the fourth type of *pranayam*.

And what is the effect of all this *pranayam*?

Tatah kshiyate prakaasha aavaranam.

They thin down the curtain around the light. *You* are the light, but you do not know this because there is a thick curtain around you; an iron curtain. *Pranayama* thins down that curtain, and makes you more transparent so that you are able to see that you are the light. *Tatah kshiyate prakaasha aavaranam* - the benefits of *pranayam*.

And then there is another benefit,

Dhaaranaasu cha yogyataa manasaha.

The mind develops this ability to stay at any one point in the body; to stay on any one thing. It gains the ability to intend. Until then, there had been no intention. You were just like a moving cloud. You had no intention at all. Now with *pranayama*, there is clarity and you are able to have an intention and a direction. That is why you will notice, after a good *pranayam*, your mind is clearer, steadier and calmer. You are able to feel your body. You are able to even meditate.

Swa vishayaa samprayoge chittaswaroopa anukaara iva indriyanaam pratyaaharaha.

The Mind is used to clinging to objects of the senses. Guided meditations give it something different to cling to. This is called *pratyaahara* - a substitute food for the mind. It is a substitution for the mind in order to coax it to come inside.

You may have danced. It was a substitution for something that you normally do. And after the dance, you felt that it was wonderful. So, it is called *pratyaahara*, a substitute for the mind to dive into.

Tatah parama vashyataa indriyaanaam.

This brings all our senses, our body and everything else together as one whole. You feel you are one whole. After a good meditation, you feel that you are whole; that you are total.

That is why Jesus said that He had come to make man whole; a complete person. That is what you feel when you do *Kriya* and when you sing in a *Satsang*. Your energy becomes full and you feel total. You become whole.

Tatah parama vashyataa indriyaanaam. Then, all your senses listen to you. You don't have to listen to them.

Parama vashyataa – you will feel much contentment, much peace and much joy. You will feel such elevation, and such completeness.

This is the effect of *pratyaahara*.

The Art of Living
&
The International Association for Human Values

Transforming Lives

The Founder

His Holiness Sri Sri Ravi Shankar

His Holiness Sri Sri Ravi Shankar is a universally revered spiritual and humanitarian leader. His vision of a violence-free, stress-free society through the reawakening of human values has inspired millions to broaden their spheres of responsibility and work towards the betterment of the world. Born in 1956 in southern India, Sri Sri was often found deep in meditation as a child. At the age of four, astonishes his teachers by reciting the Bhagavad Gita, an ancient Sanskrit scripture. He has always had the unique gift of presenting the deepest truths in the simplest of words.

Sri Sri established the Art of Living, an educational and humanitarian Non-Governmental Organisation that works in special consultative status with the Economic and Social Council (ECOSOC) of the United Nations in 1981. Present in over 140 countries, it formulates and implements lasting solutions to conflicts and issues faced by individuals, communities and nations. In 1997, he founded the International Association for Human Values (IAHV) to foster human values and lead sustainable development projects. Sri Sri has reached out to an estimated 300 million people worldwide through personal interactions, public events, teachings, Art of Living workshops and humanitarian initiatives. He has brought to the masses ancient practices which were traditionally kept exclusive, and has designed many self development techniques which can easily be integrated into daily life to calm the mind and instill confidence and enthusiasm. One of Sri Sri's most unique offerings to the world is the Sudarshan Kriya, a powerful breathing technique that facilitates physical, mental, emotional and social well-being.

Numerous honours have been bestowed upon Sri Sri, including the Order of the Pole Star (the highest state honour in Mongolia), the Peter the Great Award (Russian Federation), the Sant Shri Dnyaneshwara World Peace Prize (India) and the Global Humanitarian Award (USA). Sri Sri has addressed several international forums, including the United Nations Millennium World Peace Summit (2000), the World Economic Forum (2001, 2003) and several parliaments across the globe.

The Art of Living
In Service Around The World

(www.artofliving.org)

The largest volunteer-based network in the world, with a wide range of social, cultural and spiritual activities, the Art of Living has reached out to over 20 million people from all walks of life, since 1982. A non-profit, educational, humanitarian organization, it is committed to creating peace from the level of the individual upwards, and fostering human values within the global community. Currently, the Art of Living service projects and educational programmes are carried out in over 140 countries. The organisation works in special consultative status with the Economic and Social Council (ECOSOC) of the United Nations, participating in a variety of committees and activities related to health and conflict resolution.

The Art of Living Stress Elimination Programmes

Holistic Development of Body, Mind & Spirit The Art of Living programmes are a combination of the best of ancient wisdom and modern science. They cater to every age group - children, youth, adults -and every section of society – rural communities, governments, corporate houses, etc. Emphasizing holistic living and personal self-development, the programmes facilitate the complete blossoming of an individual's full potential. The cornerstone of all our workshops is the Sudarshan Kriya, a unique, potent breathing practice.

- The Art of Living Course Part I
- The Art of Living Course Part II
- Sahaj Samadhi Meditation
- Divya Samaaj ka Nirmaan (DSN)
- The All Round Training in Excellence
(ART Excel)
- The Youth Empowerment Seminar (YES)
(for 15-18 year olds)
- The Youth Empowerment Seminar Plus (YES+)
(for 18+ year olds)
- The Prison Programme
- Achieving Personal Excellence Program (APEX)
www.apexprogram.org
- Sri Sri Yoga www.srisriyoga.in

The International Association for Human Values

(www.iahv.org)

The International Association for Human Values (IAHV) was founded in Geneva in 1997, to foster, on a global scale, a deeper understanding of the values that unite us as a single human community. Its vision is to celebrate distinct traditions and diversity, while simultaneously creating a greater understanding and appreciation of our many shared principles. To this end, the IAHV develops and promotes programmes that generate awareness and encourage the practice of human values in everyday life. It upholds that the incorporation of human values into all aspects of life, will ultimately lead to harmony amidst diversity, and the development of a more peaceful, just and sustainable world. The IAHV works in collaboration with partners dedicated to similar goals, including governments, multilateral agencies, educational institutions, NGOs, corporations and individuals.

Service Projects

• Sustainable Rural Development

• Organic Farming

• Trauma Relief

• Peace Initiatives

• Education (www.ssrvm.org)

• Women Empowerment

• Drug Addiction Rehabilitation

International Centres

INDIA
21st KM, Kanakapura Road, Udayapura,
Bangalore – 560 082.
Karnataka.
Telephone : +91-80-67262626/27/28/29
Email : info@vvmvp.org

CANADA
13 Infinity Road
St. Mathieu du Parc
Quebec G0x 1n0
Telephone : +819- 532-3328
Fax : +819-532-2033
Email : artdevivre@artofliving.org

GERMANY
Bad Antogast 1
D - 77728 Oppenau.
Telephone : +49 7804-910 923
Fax : +49 7804-910 924
Email : artofliving.germany@t-online.de

www.srisriravishankar.org
www.artofliving.org
www.iahv.org
www.5h.org

Other titles published by Arktos:

Beyond Human Rights
by Alain de Benoist

Carl Schmitt Today
by Alain de Benoist

Manifesto for a European Renaissance
by Alain de Benoist & Charles Champetier

The Problem of Democracy
by Alain de Benoist

Germany's Third Empire
by Arthur Moeller van den Bruck

The Arctic Home in the Vedas
by Bal Gangadhar Tilak

Revolution from Above
by Kerry Bolton

The Fourth Political Theory
by Alexander Dugin

Hare Krishna in the Modern World
by Graham Dwyer & Richard J. Cole

Fascism Viewed from the Right
by Julius Evola

Metaphysics of War
by Julius Evola

Notes on the Third Reich
by Julius Evola

The Path of Cinnabar
by Julius Evola

Archeofuturism
by Guillaume Faye

Convergence of Catastrophes
by Guillaume Faye

Why We Fight
by Guillaume Faye

The WASP Question
by Andrew Fraser

We are Generation Identity
by Generation Identity

War and Democracy
by Paul Gottfried

The Saga of the Aryan Race
by Porus Homi Havewala

Homo Maximus
by Lars Holger Holm

The Owls of Afrasiab
by Lars Holger Holm

De Naturae Natura
by Alexander Jacob

Fighting for the Essence
by Pierre Krebs

Can Life Prevail?
by Pentti Linkola

Guillaume Faye and the Battle of Europe
by Michael O'Meara

New Culture, New Right
by Michael O'Meara

The National Rifle Aassociation and the Media
by Brian Anse Patrick

The Ten Commandments of Propaganda
by Brian Anse Patrick

Morning Crafts
by Tito Perdue

A Handbook of Traditional Living
by Raido

The Agni and the Ecstasy
by Steven J. Rosen

The Jedi in the Lotus
by Steven J. Rosen

It Cannot Be Stormed
by Ernst von Salomon

The Outlaws
by Ernst von Salomon

The Dharma Manifesto
by Sri Dharma Pravartaka Acharya

Celebrating Silence
by Sri Sri Ravi Shankar

Know Your Child
by Sri Sri Ravi Shankar

Management Mantras
by Sri Sri Ravi Shankar

Patanjali Yoga Sutras
by Sri Sri Ravi Shankar

Secrets of Relationships
by Sri Sri Ravi Shankar

Tradition & Revolution
by Troy Southgate

Against Democracy and Equality
by Tomislav Sunic

Nietzsche's Coming God
by Abir Taha

Generation Identity
by Markus Willinger

The Initiate: Journal of Traditional Studies
by David J. Wingfield (ed.)

CPSIA information can be obtained
at www.ICGtesting.com
Printed in the USA
BVHW071720310321
603806BV00007B/768